Intermittent Fasting

2 Books in 1: The Best Intermittent Fasting Diet + The Easy Intermittent Fasting for Women

Susan Johnson

Table Of Contents

The Best Intermittent Fasting Diet

The Easy Intermittent Fasting for Women

The Best Intermittent Fasting Diet

The Complete Beginner's Guide to Intermittent Fasting for Weight Loss, Curing the Weight Problems, and Reversing Chronic Diseases

By

Susan Johnson

Regardless, there are zero scenarios where the original author or the Publisher can be deemed liable in any fashion for any damages or hardships that may result from any of the information discussed herein.

Additionally, the information in the following pages is intended only for informational purposes and should thus be thought of as universal. As befitting its nature, it is presented without assurance regarding its continued validity or interim quality. Trademarks that are mentioned are done without written consent and can in no way be considered an endorsement from the trademark holder.

Introduction

Thank you for downloading *"The Best Intermittent Fasting Diet: The Complete Beginner's Guide to Intermittent Fasting for Weight Loss, Cure the Weight Problem, and Reverse Chronic Diseases While Enjoying!"* Many books written on intermittent fasting tend to have very vague or non-helpful information. However, this book will definitely help you learn more. Here, we will talk about every single aspect related to following intermittent fasting and explain how certain eating habits will help you gain more from it.

You have to realize that intermittent fasting can be a complicated diet regimen to understand, but once you manage to learn the ins and outs of this diet, then there is no going back. As soon as you learn how it works, your life will be very enjoyable as living a healthier life will be one less thing to worry about. Intermittent fasting is one of the most adaptive "diets" out there as you can time it however you want. Overall, intermittent fasting is the most suggested choice for people looking for a sustained healthy eating pattern.

If you are looking to enjoy life while maintaining a healthy lifestyle, then you need to understand the ins and outs of intermittent fasting. As you read this book, you will know why it is the best sustainable "diet" out there. With that being said, we should now get into the meat and potatoes of this book! Hope you enjoy it, and if you do, then make sure you follow every single tip and trick listed here!

Chapter 1: Understanding the Concept Behind Intermittent Fasting

Now, before we can truly understand what intermittent fasting is, we need to discuss what intermittent fasting truly entails. Intermittent fasting is when followers of this eating pattern are not eating for a sustained amount of time, and are eating in the eating window they have been provided — making intermittent fasting more of a cyclical eating pattern as compared to a diet. There are several ways of following the intermittent fasting diet, most of them being fulfilled within 24 hours.

The most popular fasting protocol is known as the 16/8 method, where you fast for 16 hours and eat for eight hours. In 16 hours of fasting, you are allowed to drink water or anything which has no calories to it. You are also allowed to sleep during the fasting window, which is why most people tend to stop eating later in the day to make their fast easier. As long as you follow the 16 hours of fasting and 8 hours of eating window, then there will be no issues with your protocol, and you can pick whatever time you like.

One more thing which makes fasting more user-friendly to most is the fact that there are eating restrictions, meaning you can eat whatever your heart desires within your fasting window, which makes this eating pattern very versatile when compared to a regular diet. All in all, if you are looking a change in your diet and/or eating pattern, there will be no better way to do so than intermittent fasting.

"How popular is intermittent fasting?"

Since you are reading this book, then chances are, you know how popular intermittent fasting is. Many professional doctors and fitness professionals stand by this eating pattern, making intermittent fasting one of the most popular eating patterns out there when compared to others.

Furthermore, many celebrities follow this diet to get ready for movies. Did you know that Hugh Jackman, who played Wolverine, used this awesome eating pattern to achieve his physical condition? Well, now you do! There are multiple celebrities and big names following intermittent fasting to further their goals and achievements in the fitness and health realm, which makes intermittent fasting very popular amongst the health and fitness community.

The best part is that intermittent fasting is becoming more significant day by day. Every day, there is someone on YouTube talking about their success story with intermittent fasting, or there is a new study showing how intermittent fasting can help reduce the risk of a specific disease. The way it is looking from our end, intermittent fasting will become the new way of lowering the risk of many diseases and to drop body fat within a record time without making it taxing on your body.

Since you now know how favored intermittent fasting is by many health professionals and celebrities, this should tell you that it works, and very well, at that. If you are someone who is on the fence, then this should help you change your mind.

The Science Behind Intermittent Fasting

Intermittent fasting has a lot of science to back up its many claims, but we will talk about how intermittent fasting works on a human body scientifically. You see, we have the ability to eat food whenever we want, which was not the case back when our ancestors were alive; they would sometimes go without food for days.

During that time, ancestors would use the stored fat for energy, which would lead them to survive during the days when they didn't have food. Fast forward to our generation in which we don't have to wait for food, our body stores fat and never uses it. When you are not eating for a prolonged period, your body will use its stored fat for energy.

As you know, it is not healthy to have too much fat stored as it can lead to hosts of problems and diseases. What intermittent fasting does is that it puts your body in a "starvation mode" where it uses up all the glycogen in your bloodstream and the fat stored in your body. This, as you know, is a very healthy thing for our body to get rid of excess glycogen in our blood as it leads to hosts of benefits. This is basically how intermittent fasting works in your body. Later on in this book, we will talk about how your body works to eliminate many illnesses when fasted for an extended amount of time.

Intermittent Fasting: "Why does your gut matter?"

Having a healthy gut is very important, if you are not aware. Your stomach and your brain function together, which makes your gut not only crucial for better digestion but also brain function. If you did not know, intermittent fasting could help you tremendously with fixing and helping your stomach stay healthy. The way it works is that your body gets a break from digesting all this food, and when it gets that break, it starts to clean out your gut.

Many people don't know this, but your intestine will eventually begin to collect debris, which will lead to it not functioning at its optimal rate. You see, once you stop eating, your body will start to get rid of its debris once you give it a break from digesting. Not only will this help you absorb your food at a much better rate once you do eat it, but it will also help you to have a better functioning brain.

You can read many articles on how your brain and gut are related as we will not go into further details on it, but know that you need to have better gut health overall. Because it will help you get rid of many illness and diseases, when you drink enough water and follow intermittent fasting, it becomes one of the best ways to clean out your gut. If you want better brain function and digestion, then you need to start following intermittent fasting.

How Intermittent Fasting Combats Heart Problems

As you might know, heart disease is one of the biggest killers when it comes to conditions. Intermittent fasting has also been shown to reduce the risk of heart diseases; the way it works is pretty simple. Intermittent fasting reduces the levels of LDL, which leads to heart attacks. Intermittent fasting has also been shown to lower blood pressure levels, and high blood pressure is also one of the many reasons why people tend to have heart complications.

There are many other fitness experts and professional doctors claiming that intermittent fasting works to reduce the risk of heart diseases. Even though there have been studies to back these claims up, they were done on animals. To confirm these claims, we need to make sure that these studies have been backed up with human studies.

Nonetheless, there is still some considerable evidence to follow intermittent fasting if your goal is to reduce the risk of heart diseases. One way intermittent fasting can help you to reduce the risk of heart diseases is by lowering the amount of sugar present in your bloodstream, and this has been shown to decrease the risk of heart diseases in humans, making it a plus point of intermittent fasting. So, if you are looking to lower the risk of heart diseases in the best way possible without following any diets, then intermittent fasting is the answer for you. But make sure you consult with your physician before you start any plan.

Intermittent Fasting and Insulin

Intermittent fasting plays a massive role in how your insulin is produced. When you are eating food, your insulin tends to spike up and down, resulting in frequent insulin spikes. This is where intermittent fasting comes into play; what intermittent fasting does is that it keeps your insulin stable, therefore keeping it stable throughout the day. More specifically, intermittent fasting keeps your insulin from not spiking up at all, which will help you become more insulin-sensitive.

It is crucial that you have insulin sensitivity as it will help you reduce the risk of diabetes and many other diseases related to having higher levels of insulin. But the best thing that comes with having higher insulin sensitivity is the fact that you digest food a lot better. The more insulin-sensitive you are, the better chances of you absorbing the food and converting it into energy, as compared to when you are not that insulin-sensitive; you will most likely store it into your fat reserves. With that said, it is essential that you have better insulin sensitivity for overall health.

Intermittent fasting affects your insulin in a very positive way, so make sure that you are using this tool, as it will increase insulin sensitivity in your body. Make sure that you give intermittent fasting a try, as it will help you become more insulin-sensitive and also lower the risk of many diseases such as diabetes.

The Benefits of Intermittent Fasting

As you know, there are plenty of benefits when it comes to intermittent fasting. There are not only health benefits, but there are also some mental health benefits which might interest you. Let's talk about some of the health benefits related to intermittent fasting. The main benefit which you will notice once you start following this eating protocol is the ability to lose body fat at a rapid level.

The truth is that many people can lose body fat with the help of intermittent fasting, and the best thing about it is that you really don't have to change your diet; just don't eat during the fasting window. Another benefit related to intermittent fasting is the ability to rejuvenate your cells. This process is also known as autophagy, meaning that you will slow your aging process, which to me sounds like a benefit I need! Intermittent fasting can also help you detoxify your digestive system.

As you know, you are not eating for an extended period when intermittently fasting. Therefore, you will give your intestine a break and help you resolve any issues or problems related to digestion, thus resulting in better absorption when you do eat; allowing you to absorb all the nutrients provided to your body. Intermittent fasting has been shown to increase mental focus. As there are no studies to back it up, it has only been noticed by the followers of this eating protocol, so you may or may not notice it. Overall, there are many benefits to intermittent fasting, and we will talk more about them later on in this book.

"How effective is intermittent fasting?"

Since you know the benefits to intermittent fasting, let's talk about how effective intermittent fasting can be. First of all, if your goal is to lose body fat, then there is no better way to go about it rather than to follow intermittent fasting. Many experts suggest that intermittent fasting can be of great use when you are looking to lose weight, and this is not just saying it; many users can back up those claims. Another thing that makes intermittent fasting effective is the ability to be more consistent.

When you have no diet restrictions, it becomes very easy for users to become more consistent. The more consistent you become with dieting, the more you see and experience tremendous results. This is also one of the reasons why intermittent fasting is a very effective way to lose body fat or achieve health and fitness goals. After you put all of these into consideration, you will notice that intermittent fasting is one of the most effective methods of losing fat, getting healthier, and staying more consistent with your diet. There is no consistent way around if you want your plan to be more effective. Just make sure you follow this plan to the tee if you want to see amazing effective results.

"Why you should follow intermittent fasting?"

Since you now know the importance of intermittent fasting, it all boils down to the question of how vital intermittent fasting is to your health and why you should consider it. Since we have spoken about the many benefits of intermittent fasting, it is a no-brainer that intermittent fasting can help you with a lot of things. Intermittent fasting can help you lose body fat, have better gut health, lower the risk of heart diseases, and lower the risk of diabetes, which is one of the reasons why you should consider this type of diet. Also, intermittent fasting helps you with the ability to think a lot better.

Once you start intermittent fasting, your mind will clear up, and therefore, you'll be able to think a lot better at your work or anything that you are doing which involves mental focus. One simple reason why you should consider intermittent fasting is that it keeps you more consistent. As we talked about before, consistency is the key to success in anything. The way intermittent fasting keeps you more consistent is by giving you loads of freedom, which will actually help you stay more consistent for a long time. If you want to see long-term results, then you should follow intermittent fasting. This will give you all the benefits you need and help you be more consistent.

Chapter 2: Factors to Success

In this chapter, we will discuss all the main factors you need to consider if you are looking to have better success with intermittent fasting, as many people might still find it challenging. Just remember that everyone works on their pace, so don't beat yourself to it. Moreover, in this chapter, we will show you all the little things you can start implementing towards your fasting journey and hopefully make it a much smoother experience for you.

How is Intermittent Fasting Different

You have to realize that intermittent fasting is very different when compared to the most diets out there. The reason is that intermittent fasting is more of an eating pattern rather than a diet, hence making it very different than a normal diet. This means it could be easier or harder for you; it ultimately depends on you.

Now, to get more specific on how intermittent fasting is different than other diets, let's first look at the instructions. When you're following the intermittent fasting diet, you are not restricted from eating any food. Some people eat whatever they want but still see the results such as losing body fat and feeling healthier overall while following intermittent fasting. Having the freedom to eat whatever you want is one of the significant differrences between a normal diet and intermittent fasting.

Another difference between normal and intermittent fasting is the eating window. Many people aren't aware of the fact that when following most diets, you have to eat every two hours, as compared to intermittent fasting where you don't eat for 12 hours to 48 hours depending on the person. Doing this makes it very different from a normal diet, so make sure you are aware of the differences which come along with intermittent fasting.

Picking the Right Fasting Protocol

Picking the right fasting protocol is one of the most crucial things to consider before you start intermittent fasting. This is where most people make the mistake of choosing the wrong intermittent fasting protocol. This is also why you need to understand all the protocols provided and then make an educated decision on which one fits your lifestyle and your goals. In later chapters, we will discuss the different main types of intermittent fasting protocols.

But for now, let's briefly talk about the protocols and which one you should be picking based on your lifestyle and goals. Now, there are two main types of intermittent fasting. The first one is the one-day fast: this is where you fast for 12 to 16 hours, and you eat for 12 to 8 hours during that day. This fasting method is ideal for people who are looking to lose weight and still see the health benefits related to intermittent fasting. There have been many studies showing that following a similar type of fasting protocol has shown to lower the risk of heart diseases and diabetes — giving this protocol an excellent balance for someone looking to get the health benefits alongside the aesthetic benefits.

The second protocol is strictly for people who are looking to lose body fat. This is following a protocol which includes one whole day of fasting; many people observe this fasting protocol by fasting for one day and eating normally the next day. This puts them in a 20-25% calorie deficit, therefore, optimizing them for fat loss. If your goal is to lose fat and only that, then I strictly suggest that you follow the fasting protocol similar to this. In later chapters, we will discuss more the two types of fasting protocols so that you will have a better idea of how these work.

Ease into Fasting

The problem with intermittent fasting is that most people start intermittent fasting abruptly. You have to realize that intermittent fasting is very foreign to your body as of right now; meaning, for you to be successful with intermittent fasting, you need to take it step-by-step. More specifically, you need to ease into it. Let's talk about some things you can do to ease into intermittent fasting. The first thing you need to do is start with a more natural fast. Instead of jumping straight into 24-hour fasting, you should consider skipping meals first or doing a 12-hour fast.

Easing into intermittent fasting is the best way to ensure that you see optimal results, so if you feel like fasting for 12 hours is too much for you in the beginning, then perhaps start skipping a meal and then slowly build up to a 12-hour fast. Many people have tried intermittent fasting cold turkey, and they have failed miserably; so please, do not overlook the idea of intermittent fasting step-by-step and easing into it. Just start with whatever feels easy for you, and depending on individuals, it could be starting by skipping one meal or merely starting with a 12-hour fast. But whatever you decide to start with, make sure it feels easy for you in the beginning.

The Hunger Pangs

Many of you might have heard of hunger pangs, and it is when you feel pain in your stomach from the lack of calorie consumption. This is quite common when intermittently fasting, especially in the beginning when your body is not used to eating so little throughout the day. Some might notice hunger pangs when intermittently fasting, so there are some ways to avoid them, which we will talk about now.

The first way to prevent it is drinking more water. What water does is help you stay hydrated throughout the day and reduce the risk of hunger pangs. Moreover, water will help you stay feeling full for a more extended period. If the hunger pain gets too excessive, consider chewing gum. This will trick your body into thinking that you're eating food when you're really not.

Please use this technique when the pain gets extremely unbearable. If you can try, avoid chewing gum as it can break your fast. Other than these two techniques, there isn't much to do if you want to prevent hunger pangs. Just know that it will subside the longer you follow intermittent fasting, and some of you might not even notice it as this is more of a heads-up than anything.

Drink Lots of Water

When you're intermittent fasting, the best thing you can do for the body is to drink a lot of water. Many people know that water is beneficial to humans and contains no calories at all, which is why it makes it a great idea to drink a lot of water while intermittent fasting. When you drink, more water while intermittent fasting, you will feel a lot less hungry. Another good thing it will do is also help you clear out any toxins in your body.

When you're fasting for an extended period, you detoxify your body and water will help you detoxify it even further. This is why drinking water during and after you break your fast is crucial. Another reason why you should drink more water during your fast is that you want to ensure that you don't get any hunger pangs, as you know that when you drink water, your chances of hunger pangs will reduce significantly.

Overall, it is in your best interest to drink more water, so go ahead and have some to avoid many severe side effects that you might face in the beginning and detoxify your body even further when fasting. However, it is most important to suppress appetite so that you don't break your fast when you don't need to.

How Not to Binge

When your fast, you will have many cravings to start binging on every food you see. Therefore, it is very critical that you don't indulge in your desires and start binging. This is why we need to talk about this subject. There are many ways to stop yourself from binge eating, but we will talk about the most common ones out there and perhaps help you not indulge in those cravings.

The first way to ensure that you don't start binging during your fast is to ensure that you are hydrated. As you know, keeping yourself hydrated actually suppresses your appetite, and therefore, it will cause you to feel a lot less hungry throughout the day. Another way to ensure that you don't binge is to drink coffee and tea during the fast. The good thing about coffee and tea is that there are no calories when drunk with no milk or sugar. So during your fast, if you start consuming some coffee or tea, it will actually suppress your appetite and even give you some energy; which makes this a great idea to be consuming.

When fasting, if you want some energy and you want to suppress your appetite, make sure you drink a lot of coffee throughout the day while fasting. When I say a lot, I mean two cups to three cups of day, and no more than that. Nonetheless, make sure you're following these methods to suppress your appetite and to ensure that you stay on track with your intermittent fasting.

Eating Healthy and Nutritious Meals

Eating healthy nutritious meals is very important if your goal is to lose weight. However, it is imperative that you eat healthy when you're intermittently fasting and you're looking to lose weight and live a healthier life. Even though intermittent fasting allows you to eat whatever you want and still see the results are you looking for, it is in your best interest to start eating healthy when you break your fast.

This is strictly personal opinion based on experience. Many health experts will not agree with me on this, but here are my two cents: the reason why you need to be eating healthy and having nutritious meals is to take your goals to the next level. When you start eating healthy in conjunction with fasting, magic starts to happen.

It's like a cherry on top if you are going to lose 10 lbs. by merely fasting and not changing your diet. Well then, intermittent fasting and diet in conjunction will help you lose 20 lbs., and at the same time, you'll lose 10 pounds while eating whatever you want to. Do you see what I'm trying to say? If you want good results, simply follow intermittent fasting, but if you wish to look at terrific results to eating healthy and nutritious meals while intermittent fasting, these are just aesthetic benefits.

Once you start eating healthy and nutritious food, your health will get a lot better as well. In conjunction with intermittent fasting, you will detoxify your body and organs, making your body healthy.

Keep a Journal

Keeping a journal is a great idea; this will help you stay more motivated in the process of intermittent fasting. Write down everything that you're feeling and doing, and build off that. When you journal your thoughts and feelings, you will be able to control them a lot better as this will help you understand when you feel and how to deal with your feelings. Many successful people journal their thoughts and feelings, and it is one of the ways to ensure optimal success. Simply get a book and start writing everything from how you were feeling and how you are dealing with your issues. Whenever you start feeling similar matters on a following day, simply go back to your journal and read how you dealt with it.

Also, every month, make sure you recap how consistent you were with your diet and fasting, and try to do better the next month. These are the main reasons why I recommend carrying a journal, so go ahead and start journaling.

Get Rid of the Nay-sayers

There will be many non-supporters that you will encounter after you start your journey of intermittent fasting. Make sure that you stay away from these toxic people. It doesn't matter how close you are with them; they will always try and bring you down when you try to do something better for yourself. They want you to do well, but they never want you to do better than them, so make sure that you surround yourself with positive people and well-wishers.

Make sure that you're around people who teach you rather than bring you down; and if you can find them, it is best that you keep your intermittent fasting goals and lifestyle to yourself and not talk about it in front of the people as they will only bring you down. Just be aware that there will be some negativity coming from friends and family – just ignore it and focus on yourself.

Stay on Track for 30 Days

This is perhaps one of the most important things to take home: if you can stick around for 30 days, you will see amazing results for an extended period. Here's the thing: it takes approximately 21 to 40 days to create a habit. Meaning, if you can keep fasting for at least 30 days, it will become second nature to you, and you can keep fasting and see amazing results day-by-day. This is also where the journal comes in: make sure that you are journaling every day for 30 days as this will help you stay on track. Do whatever you can to stay on track for 30 days.

Once intermittent fasting becomes a habit for you, then there is no stopping you. Journal every day; make sure you're doing everything you can to avoid breaking your fast for 30 days, like drinking more water, coffee, or tea. Once you have managed to do that, you can perhaps get into more intense fasting. As your body gets used to it, you will start being able to keep going with it. Keep that in mind when you first start your fasting.

An Important Thing to Consider

There aren't a lot of important things to consider as we have discussed most of them. However, let's talk about the most common mistakes you will make and the health risks involved with intermittent fasting. If you're pregnant or trying to conceive, then intermittent fasting is not for you. Please do not intermittently fast if you're pregnant or trying to conceive as it can cause miscarriage.

Also, if you are not used to intermittent fasting at all, then you need to start slow. There have been many cases of people fainting on the first day they start intermittent fasting; this is simply because they're not used to it. So, make sure that you take it slow. Start with meal-skipping, then get into a 12-hour fast; after that, perhaps you can go further from there. Make sure that you follow the 12-hour fast for at least three weeks before you lengthen your fasting periods.

Finally, the main thing to consider when intermittently fasting is to consult with your physician or doctor. I am not a doctor, so I can't tell you if you're fit enough to intermittently fast. Make sure that you ask your doctor whether you are fit or not because if you aren't, you might experience many health issues. Just know everything before you start intermittently fasting.

Chapter 3: Why Other Diets Don't Work

Since we have talked about the benefit of eating healthy food when intermittently fasting, we will not talk about the diets you need to stay away from to achieve optimal success while intermittently fasting. There are many diets which are supposedly healthy for you even though they're really not, and unlike intermittent fasting, they're not sustainable for a long period. Nonetheless, we will talk about the main things to consider while picking out your diet regimen. Make sure you that read this chapter very carefully to achieve optimal success.

Most Diets Are not Maintainable

As you might know, many diets aren't maintainable for an extended period; the simple reason behind it is that they make you do too much in a short period, which is why we don't recommend following any type of diet when following intermittent fasting; you must merely eat healthy and nutritious food.

Although there is one diet that we think that goes well with intermittent fasting, we will talk about that diet and further details later on in this book. Nonetheless, let's talk about the reasons why most diets are not maintainable. The reason why they are not maintainable especially during intermittent fasting is that they make you undereat a lot. When you undereat because of intermittent fasting, the chances of you giving up on diets are incredibly high; don't get me wrong, being in a caloric deficit while intermittent fasting is fine, but to do it right is another thing.

There is a sweet spot between intermittent fasting and caloric deficit, if you mess that up, then the chances of you maintaining a proper eating schedule will go drastically down. It is enough to eat healthy, nutritious meals while intermittent fasting. Later on, we will discuss a diet which can actually help you lose even more body fat.

Fad Diets Can Be Harmful

You have probably seen these diets before, and they are very prominent in magazines. Stay away from fad diets as much as possible because they don't work at all and they put you in a worse position health-wise. When you are in a caloric deficit for an extended period, it can mess with your hormones, and fat loss will worsen in the long run; the worst thing is that it affects your metabolism. When you don't eat enough calories for a long period, it changes your metabolism in the long run.

Another effect that fad diets can have is the development of eating disorders. Many people don't know this, but eating disorders are some of the biggest problems people face when they follow fad diets. Depending on the fat content of the diet, a diet could be low-carb, or it may involve surviving on liquids for the rest of your days. This is not ideal for anyone looking to lose weight, so the best thing you can do is stay away from these diets and just focus on intermittent fasting.

The Yo-Yo Diet

Yo-yo dieting is when you lose weight but you go back really fast. There have been many studies that show that diets are not optimal for many people, as it slows down your metabolism, which in the long term cause you to gain more weight. Trust me that you don't want to have a yo-yo diet in the long-term.

Let's talk about a couple of things that you might be doing which could be similar to yo-yo dieting: the first sign that you might have a yo-yo diet is having too little carbs. Your body needs a certain amount of carbs throughout the day to survive, and it is needed to lose weight. You need to give your body just the right amount of carbs to put it into a caloric deficit without damaging the hormones and metabolism. If you feel incredibly sluggish throughout the day for an extended period, then you need to rethink your diet. Perhaps you need to add more carbs to diet; you must have just enough calories throughout the day to allow you to get out of the yo-yo diet cycle. Nonetheless, if you are on a yo-yo diet, you must get away from it; if you do not keep doing what you are doing, chances are, you are in a much better place.

On Eating Disorders

You may be facing eating disorders, or you may not know what eating disorders are. Eating disorders make you unable to control what you're eating or make it hard for you to eat healthy, to put in layman's term. The best way to avoid eating disorders is to stay away from yo-yo dieting and any fad diets. The good thing about intermittent fasting is that it prevents you from getting into any eating disorders as it teaches you how to control your appetite and when to eat, which are very healthy for your body. If you think that you're facing eating disorders, then talk to your doctor as they might be able to help you a lot better.

How Diets Can Make You Binge

So far, we have talked about the many reasons why many diets can put you in a very unhealthy place and cause you to binge. The reason why you binge while on a diet is that there are too many restrictions. You need to follow a diet that does not have a lot of restrictions, which can help you sustain it for an extended period of time. To reiterate, the only reason why you binge while on a diet is that there are too many restrictions. If you want to avoid binging, just pick a plan which works for you.

A Form of Starvation

Most diets are a form of starvation; the reason why is that you're not getting enough nutrients throughout the day when you follow them. Most diets don't allow you to eat enough food, and therefore, your body goes into starvation mode. A certain amount of starvation is fine, but most diets put you in a position where you don't have even enough nutrients to have a properly functioning body, which is why dieting can become a form of starvation, so try and stay away from fad diets as much as possible.

Diets Can Be Restricting

As you know, diets impose many restrictions, such as pinpointing certain food that you can't eat or imposing a limit on calories that you can consume, which is why it is imperative that you don't follow a diet; it can cause you to become more proactive towards indulging in cravings. Not only that, there are some restrictions which don't make sense at all. Most diets suggest many stupid things such as not eating solid food and surviving on liquids, which is not a great idea if you are looking towards a healthy lifestyle overall. I can keep going on my tirade about restrictions which come along with diets, but you get the point. Simply stay away from diets until you have found the right one for you.

Increased Craving When Dieting

The difference between intermittent fasting and dieting is this: when you're intermittently fasting, you actually start losing cravings for certain kinds food as compared to dieting, when you do not lose any cravings; sometimes, you gain more.

Many people gain a lot of cravings while dieting; they develop craving mostly for sugars as this is what they're missing in their diet. If you develop cravings for food that have a lot of sugar, chances are, you're not eating enough food. Moreover, you can still lose weight while eating a good amount of food; you may have noticed having cravings before if you've tried out a diet before.

These are why we recommend that you stay away from dieting. As of right now, we've just discussed all the problems related to dieting to steer you away from them. Don't get me wrong; at the beginning of intermittent fasting, you will notice many cravings for food. However, if you give it a week or two, the cravings will go away, and in fact, you will start to notice that you are in control of what you eat and when you eat.

Diets Can Cause Weight Gain

Remember how we talked about your metabolism slowing down when following a traditional type of dieting? Well, it is true. When you diet for an extended period and you lose the right amount of weight, chances are, you will gain it back rather quickly. You see, when you don't eat enough food, your metabolism will go down, and once your metabolism goes down, you will start to notice a tremendous amount of weight gain; this is why many people recommend getting off the cycle from time to time because they know that it's causing damage to their metabolism. Meaning, if you don't want to gain weight, then don't diet as you will gain it back very quickly. Your diet might have been successful for a while, but chances are, you will gain the weight back.

As we explain to you how you will gain your weight back while dieting, it is very common to see drastic weight loss. It is simply because you will be in a caloric deficit, which will put your body in starvation mode. However, once you get out of starvation mode, your body will go into hibernation mode. This is when you will store all the fat that you have for energy. Anything you eat will be used to store energy and go into your fat stores, which makes sense because your body doesn't know when it will get food again. So, make sure that you are aware of the fact that you will gain the weight back. If you happen to be successful in dieting, you'll notice that you're gaining your weight back. Then the only way you can fix it is by intermittently fasting because intermittent fasting not only raises your metabolism but keeps your body in a healthy level of starvation mode. This will make your body lose fat and maintain a healthy metabolism rate, so you won't gain your weight back ever again.

Cholesterol Norepinephrine and Epinephrine Increase

These hormones are one of the most essential hormones in your body, as they ensure that you lose weight at a specific rate. When you're dieting chances, your norepinephrine and epinephrine will increase, which is good for weight loss. However, you don't want unhealthy spikes of these hormones, as something that comes up quickly will shoot down quickly. So, be aware of the fact that when you're dieting extremely, it will go up; but once you stop it, will shoot back down.

On the other hand, when intermittent fasting, your hormone levels will increase and stabilize at the top, causing no unnecessary side effects what you might expect from dieting. Just be aware that before you start any diets, and as always, we recommend following intermittent fasting.

Your Body May Have a Problem Releasing Waste

You have to realize that your body is brilliant when it finds out that it is in a starvation mode. It will hold on to everything possible for energy, which also includes your waste. This will cause a big problem in your body if you can't release your waste correctly. There are two ways dieting affects your waist releasing. The first way is by your body holding onto your waste for energy, and the second way is by your body not getting enough nutrients or fibers to digest the food properly and turn it into waste.

There are some ways to ensure that it doesn't happen: the first way would be to ensure that you're getting enough fiber in your diet. If you want to make sure that you're getting rid of your waste correctly, then make sure your fiber intake and water intake is up there. Dieting or not, you need to make sure that fiber intake and water intake is at a healthy amount for you to get rid of your waste. Another way to ensure that your body doesn't hold on to waste is as effortless as not to diet.

Lack of Energy When Working Out

When you're not eating enough food, or I should say nutritionally dense food, then the chances of you having a great workout will drop down drastically. To ensure that you don't have bad workouts, start eating more food and, more specifically, healthy food. If you have dieted, you will know that you don't get enough nutrients in your body, and therefore, you will have a lot less energy when working out or hitting the gym.

The gym is also a big part when it comes to losing weight and staying healthy overall, which is why we recommend you to work on your body. Accordingly, this would be to ensure that you have a great workout at the gym, and you get the most out of your workouts. There are a couple of ways to do that: first, make sure you're getting enough micronutrients such as vitamins and minerals. The second way to do that is to eat enough food. Once these two things are in place, you will healthily lose weight while ensuring that you don't compromise your health.

While intermittently fasting, you will start to notice that your energy will become more abundant during your workouts, which is why it is a great idea to intermittently fasting if working out is a big part of your life. Nonetheless, the main takeaway from this is that your diet shouldn't negatively affect your workout.

Magic Weight Loss Scammers

Finally, we need to talk about the big elephant in the room – the magic weight loss scammers. You have seen them, and you already know what they are like. The best you can do is to stay away from these weight loss scammers as they don't care about anything else but your money.

A couple of ways to tell that they are magic weight loss scammers is if they make claims which are too good to be true. You might have heard the saying, "If it sounds too good to be true, it is." If you have a feeling that these weight loss scammers might be genuine, then the first thing you need to do is ask any professional or your doctor about the diet the scammers are offering.

If your doctor or your fitness expert doesn't agree with it, then chances are it is a big scam. Like we always say, do your research before you start anything, which is why we wrote this book. This is also to show you how intermittent fasting works. However, for now, your goal is to stay away from fad diets, more specifically, weight loss scammers which will do whatever it takes to get your money.

Chapter 4: Diet Nutrition, Exercise, and Rest

When following intermittent fasting, a trio of main things you need to consider are diet, exercise, and rest. In this chapter, we will go into depth on how you can ensure that all things listed above are in check. Many of you might be falling back on eat least one of these aspects, and the sooner you realize which one it is and fix it, the better.

Diet and Nutrition

In the previous chapter, we already talked about the importance of diet and nutrition. Let's further discuss it to ensure that you are optimizing this aspect as well. Having the right diet and nutrition can either make or break you in the realm of fitness and health. The simplest way to ensure that your diet and nutrition is on point is to keep it simple; by that, I mean not following any crazy diets which will hinder your goals and success.

The best way to go about it is to just to eat healthy food during your eating window. Please do not make your food intake very complicated. If your goal is to lose weight, having a little caloric deficit and eating good vegetables and meat will do the trick. This will provide you with optimal nutrition while striving you towards your goals. The reason why we keep bringing up diet and nutrition is to show you that you can follow intermittent fasting without overthinking. If your diet or nutrition plan is too complicated for you and becomes a chore, then chances are, you're not following the right strategy. The next time you're planning out your food intake, make sure that this isn't a chore for you but more of a lifestyle.

How Intermittent Fasting Affects Your Body

Intermittent fasting works uniquely, so let's talk about it. When you're following an intermittent fasting type of eating protocol, you are going into a starvation mode. When you're in starvation mode, your body thinks that it's not getting enough food, and therefore, it starts breaking down your fat stores.

The same thing happened to our ancestors; they would go without food for a couple of days, and once they did find food, they are much to store body fat so they can use it for later. We are merely following a diet which was used by our ancestors. Believe it or not, they were a lot healthier than us, and they didn't have any diseases such as diabetes and so on.

Nonetheless, let's get into the science of intermittent fasting. When you are fasting, your body will burn off all the glycogen and your bloodstreams for a couple of hours. Once it has burnt out all the glycogen in your bloodstream, it will start to use your fat stores for energy, which is where the magic happens. You will burn more fat throughout the day than you would following any other diet, which makes intermittent fasting one of the best diets to follow if your goal is to lose fat or to lower the risk of diseases.

Eating Wrong Food Can Counter Those Effects

Eating the wrong food can counter those effects during intermittent fasting. Even though when you're following intermittent fasting, you're allowed to eat whatever you want. However, that doesn't mean it is the optimal way to go about it. Here's the thing: if you want to ensure that you're not countering the effects from intermittent fasting, then you need to eat the right food.

Since you already know the right food to eat when intermittent fasting, let's talk about the food that you shouldn't eat when you're following an intermittent fasting type of protocol. The first kind of food you should not eat is anything which would be considered junk food, even though most people have seen success despite eating junk food. We don't recommend that you do the same because, chances are, you will convert that food into fat more quickly than you would while eating healthy food. Another reason why you should not eat junk food while intermittent fasting is that it would not help you lower the risk of any diseases. Even though intermittent fasting is a powerful way to reduce the risk of diseases, it can't be countered without the consumption of healthy food.

On the other hand, eating junk food by itself will increase the risk of heart diseases and diabetes. To keep everything simple, stay away from anything which would be considered fast food. Once you manage to do that, you will be in a lot better place.

Important Food Groups for Nutrition

There are many essential food groups to consider when following intermittent fasting. To keep things very simple, you must eat only the kinds of food which were available thousands of years ago. These include meats, vegetables, and some grains here and there. The thing that you need to consider to eat food which are low in the glycemic index so that you don't increase your insulin levels when you do eat those food.

When your insulin level spikes consistently, you put yourself at risk of contracting type 2 diabetes, which is why you need to research the types of food you're eating. So, make sure that whatever you're eating has a low glycemic index rating.

Most of the time, food such as brown rice, meat, and vegetables have a very low glycemic index. Meaning, they will not cause your insulin to spike very quickly, and it will take time for you to burn off those calories from the food giving you a sustained amount of energy throughout the day. This is where you want to be when following intermittent fasting, and you need to have a sustained amount of energy throughout the day.

The main three food groups of nutrition are carbohydrates, protein, and fats. It would be best if you make sure that all three of these come from good healthy food. It will help if you are more careful with your carbohydrate intake, as excessive intake of carbohydrates will spike your insulin very quickly. Simply eat carbohydrates, which are low in the glycemic index, and you will be fine.

"Do intermittent fasting and exercise go together?"

Many people feel that intermittent fasting exercise does not go together, just because you're starving yourself throughout the day. However, the truth is that when intermittently fasting, you have terrific workouts, and there's a reason behind it.

When you're intermittently fasting, your body goes into starvation mode; when your body is in starvation mode, it raises your adrenaline, which is why some people notice that they have better mental focus while fasting. When your adrenaline goes up, you have more energy to do physical tasks because your body feels like it needs to fight for food. This is why you will have a lot of energy throughout the day when you work out. From personal experience, I can tell you that I've had one of the best workouts while intermittently fasting. The best part about working out while fasting is that you will burn fat for energy instead of glycogen. Meaning, you will actually gain more benefits and lose more fat from working out while fasting. Some have said that intermittent fasting lowers their strength levels, but it should not be noticeable if you're not a powerlifter. If your goal is merely to lose weight, intermittently fasting would be the best thing to do while working out.

Go for High-Intensity Workouts After Eating

Here is the truth: the best way to burn fat while intermittently fasting is to follow a high-intensity type of workout plan. When you follow a high-intensity workout, you'll actually burn a lot more calories for an extended period. Ideally, you should be working out right after you break your fast; this will put you in a position where you have some food in you to burn off. High-intensity workouts work great when your goal is to have better cardiovascular health and to burn off some fat.

Ideally, you should be doing a cardio workout at least three to four times a week to ensure that your fat is actually melting off. Still, in conjunction, you need to make sure that your workouts are high-intensity as this will not only burn off more fat but also raise your hormones. This will help you live a better, healthier life. The next time you're planning workouts, make sure that they are high-intensity and short. This will ensure that you are getting closer to your goals every day without leaving any stones unturned.

Eat High-Protein Meals

You might have noticed that many people in the fitness industry suggest eating high-protein meals. There's a reason for that: protein is one of the best macronutrients when you're looking to burn fat and to live a healthier life. Let's get into the science as to why protein is essential when intermittently fasting.

The first thing that protein does is preserve your muscle. When you have more muscle mass in your body, you burn more fat. Therefore, it is essential to have more protein to prevent muscle loss. Another thing protein is really good for is burning off fat. Protein is the macronutrient which requires the most calories to digest, which is why we need more protein; by getting more of it, you burn more fat. Protein takes much energy to digest; energy comes from calories, and calories become fat.

Another great thing about protein is that it does not raise your insulin levels. Unlike carbohydrates, protein does not increase your insulin levels. This is why it is a great idea to have more protein in your diet because you can get energy without raising your insulin levels. If your goal is to lose weight, you will look a lot better and live a healthy life by getting protein. Thus, you need to have enough protein in your diet. Protein is a building block, and it builds muscle; it burns fat, and most importantly, it keeps you healthy for the days to come. Make sure that you are getting enough protein in your diet.

Rest

So far, we have talked about diet and working out, and the truth is that those are the most important things to consider when intermittently fasting or going on any diet, for that matter. However, the most critical thing we tend to overlook is rest. If you do not rest enough, then you will not see the results that you are looking for.

There needs to be a right balance between exercising and rest, which is what we will talk about in this section of the book. Ideally, you should be resting at least twice a week after your workouts, so you should work out no more than five times a week, and that includes your cardio and weight-training workouts. If you don't rest, your body will counteract the stimulus you are providing it with to put on muscle and lose fat. If you don't want that to happen, you should make sure that you give yourself twice a week of rest.

Another form of rest is sleep. You need to ensure that you are getting an ample amount of sleep every day; this will also help you recover from your workouts. More importantly, it will help you produce the optimal amount of hormones that you need for healthy body functions. Some people say that you need eight to ten hours of sleep, but the truth is that you can survive with six to eight hours of sleep. Just make sure that you're getting enough sleep to help your boy recover from working out and from the daily stress that you might have acquired. Overall, rest is an essential part of your fitness and health, so the last thing that you must do is to overlook it.

Chapter 5: Metabolism, Brain, Muscle Mass, Hunger, and Blood Sugar Levels

Intermittent fasting has been known to affect the body drastically, mostly in a positive manner when done correctly. In this chapter, we will get into the specifics of it all, and also show you how intermittent fasting truly affects your body inside and out.

Intermittent Fasting and Your Metabolism

Intermittent fasting has shown to raise your metabolism and has also proved to lower your metabolism, which is why you need to follow intermittent fasting the right way. Here's the thing when following intermittent fasting, you will most likely boost your metabolism in the beginning, as your body will go into starvation mode it will start to use your body fat for energy. Once it starts using body fat for energy, it will have to increase metabolism, whenever your metabolism is increased, and you will be burning more calories as we know this.

However, if you keep on with intermittent fasting for a prolonged period, your body will understand and will burn calories at a much lower rate. The reason why is because your body is brilliant, it does not want to burn up many calories when it knows that there aren't back in time soon. Hence, it slows down the process of burning calories and raising metabolism. For you to get the most benefits out of intermittent fasting, you have to become smarter more specifically to become more intelligent than your body. The way to do that is by cycling off intermittent fasting. You will see significant fat loss benefits from intermittent fasting for about 4 to 6 weeks, after that it will go downhill. Your goal should be to cycle on and off of intermittent fasting, and this will allow you to see all the benefits while not harming your metabolism.

How Fasting Can Hurt Your Metabolism

As we just briefly explained to you how intermittent fasting affects your metabolism, let's talk about how it can damage your metabolism when looking at the science. When your following intermittent fasting, you put yourself into a starvation mode. Once you're in starvation mode, your body will do anything possible to survive which means burning off any glycogen in the bloodstream and start using fat stores for energy. To use fat stores for energy, your body will need to increase metabolism; and therefore allow you to burn more fat.

Your metabolism and the number of calories you burn go hand-in-hand, which is why having high metabolism helps you burn a lot more calories. However, the thing is, your body will get used to the starvation mode and will burn a lot fewer calories once you get into it a little bit deeper. Your body is brilliant, it will only use the number of calories it needs to survive. Once it becomes acquainted with the starvation mode you put in your body in, it will become a lot more effective at burning calories and therefore lower your metabolism. If you don't follow intermittent fasting the right way, it can lead to metabolism slowing down for the rest of your life. Make sure you're following intermittent fasting the right way, and by cycling on and off.

Fasting and Brain

Many CEOs and successful people follow intermittent fasting because of the effects it has on the brain. Even though it has not been scientifically proven, intermittent fasting has shown to increase brain function allowing you to have more focus throughout the day to get the work done. When you're intermittent fasting, your body becomes a lot more focused because it feels like it needs to be hunting to get more food.

Which is simply the Primal inmate in us, when you're hunting you need to be focused on getting the kill which is why when you're in the starvation mode you become a lot more focused. From personal experience I can tell you that intermittent fasting is helping my mental function and focus while doing anything, even driving a car while intermittent fasting has made me a lot more focus on the road.

The hormone which is released while you are intermittent fasting is known as your adrenaline hormone. Your adrenaline is a lot higher when intermittent fasting when your adrenaline is high you're in a flight or fight situation. This is when your body will do anything's possible, to make sure that you're focused and do what you have to do. The adrenal hormone was more used by our ancestors not to get killed by predators. In the modern day, we use hormone for work-related stuff or anything which requires mental focus.

Burns Fat for Fuel

You will burn a lot more calories following intermittent fasting than you would following any diet out there. Most diets out there, make you eat 5 to 6 times a day every 2 to 3 hours. The reason why it won't work is that your glycogen will always be full and therefore your body will be using glycogen for energy and not be using its fat store. Here's the thing your body needs to be in the starvation mode to use fat stores, but your body is very smart, it will not use body fat stores if it does not need to.

What intermittent fasting does as I said is put you into starvation mode, once you're in starvation mode your body will use the fat for energy. Once your body starts using fat for energy, it will burn off the fat stores that you have giving you a more aesthetically pleasing physique. The reason why your body will be using the fat stored glycogen is because you will not be providing your body glycogen for a long time, when you don't give your body glycogen for an extended period of time the only way it will function properly is to use the fat stores that you have in your body.

Another reason why intermittent fasting helps you burn more fat is that it puts you into ketosis. This is when your body will strictly use fat for energy and not glycogen. In later chapters, we will talk about how specific diets can help you burn more fat while following intermittent fasting. However, for now, know that intermittent fasting will help you burn more fat than glycogen throughout the day.

Boost Your Energy

Remember how we said intermittent fasting boost your adrenaline, which is one of the reasons why you will have more energy while intermittent fasting. When you have high amounts of adrenaline and your body, you will have more energy to do physical and mental tasks. Another way intermittent fasting helps you boost your energy is by not giving you any ups and downs in your insulin level.

Have you ever had the feeling of overeating food and feeling very tired right after? The reason you feel exhausted right after is that your insulin is spiking up to digest the food. When your insulin spikes up, you'll feel lethargy and tiredness. When intermittent fasting you will have no insulin spikes during your fast, which will allow you to have a sustained amount of energy throughout the day and therefore boosting power. These two things in combination will help your energy tremendously while intermittent fasting. Which is why intermittent fasting raises your energy, and when you mix it up with working out then you are set on the part of excellent energy level throughout the day.

Boost Human Growth Hormone (HGH) Levels

Intermittent fasting has shown to increase human growth hormone levels tremendously, let's get into the science how this works. When you're intermittent fasting, your body will not be producing insulin or spiking sporadically throughout the day, which is one of the reasons why your human growth hormone will go up.

The thing is growth hormone, and Insulin cannot coexist, technically they can but if your insulin is spiking up your growth hormone will be going down and vice versa. To explain it at layman's term, since your insulin won't be spiking up sporadically throughout the day your growth hormone will be going out gradually. When you mix it up with your working out routine, this will be a great way to increase your growth hormone.

There have been studies showing that intermittent fasting has increased growth hormone by up to four thousand percent, which is insane if you think about it. Growth hormone has many benefits including more muscle mass, a higher rate of fat loss and the best of them all anti-aging effects. Meaning if these benefits sound useful to you, then you need to follow intermittent fasting and moreover make sure your insulin is in check.

Muscle Mass and Intermittent Fasting Hunger

Many people who follow intermittent fasting, feel like they will lose muscle while following the eating protocol. However, the truth is they won't lose any muscle at all, and instead, they will gain a lot more muscle since their growth hormone will be going up.

Here's The thing, for you to lose muscle while intermittent fasting you will have to fast for more than 3 days to see some loss. There have been studies showing that 48 Hours of fasting has had no effects on muscle loss. So, if you're thinking about not following intermittent fasting because you might lose your muscle, then don't because you won't lose your muscle while following intermittent fasting. Actually, intermittent fasting is better for fat loss and helps you gain more muscle. Here's why. As was mentioned, intermittent fasting has shown to increase growth hormone levels, growth hormone levels have also proved to increase muscle mass. Put two and two together you see a recipe to more muscle and less fat.

Now that we've discussed muscle mass and intermittent fasting, let's briefly touch upon hunger you might experience while following intermittent fasting. For the first couple of weeks, he will notice some Hunger while fasting. It is incredibly reasonable to feel that way, just because your body is not used to intermittent fasting. Give it a couple of weeks, and you should be in a routine of intermittent fasting and not feeling of hunger.

Balancing Hunger While Fasting

Balancing hunger while fasting, is very easy to do later on in the stage. Although in the beginning, it would be tough for you to manage your hunger, there are some ways to avoid that, and we will show you how to do that. The first thing would be to start intermittent fasting slowly, and you need to make sure that intermittent fasting has been eased into because you don't want to give up midway while fasting. Perhaps starting with a skipping meal type of fasting or anything which seems natural to you is something you should start with. Another way to ensure that you don't notice any hunger while fasting is to make sure that you are drinking plenty of water.

There have been studies showing that when you drink more water suppresses your appetite, so make sure you're drinking much water during and after you're fast. The last one you can suppress hunger while fasting or balance it. I should say it is to make sure that you drink more coffee and tea throughout the day. Not only will coffee and tea give you a lot more energy, but it would also help you to balance out your hunger. Coffee and tea have been shown to reduce hunger levels, merely have a couple of coffee throughout the day. Just make sure that there are no additives for the coffee, as we don't want to break her fast so I can see me something that has calories in them.

Eating Enough to Break Your Fast

The truth is that you need to make sure that you are getting enough before you break your fast, the best way to do that is to count your calories. Counting calories isn't as hard as you think it is, the reason why it isn't so hard is there many tools you can use online to make sure that you're getting enough calories throughout the day. What intermittent fasting does merely allows you to eat at a particular time of the day. It tricks your body into thinking that they're in starvation mode when they're not.

Nonetheless, you can still get enough calories to put on muscle lose weight or to maintain. The way to do that is to break it into two big meals since you only have a particular time to get all your calories, but the main thing you need to make sure that you are eating enough before you break your fast. To make sure they are eating enough before you break your fast is to calculate all the meals that you are going to be having during your eating window. I figure out how many calories you need for your goals, and then breaking into two meals. This will let you have enough food when you break your fast and not see any adverse effects that you might recognize from dieting. It is very common for people to undereating during intermittent fasting because they only have a specific time to eat food, make sure you're not making that mistake.

Get Some Sleep

I'm sure you know the importance of getting enough sleep throughout the day, especially when intermittent fasting you need to make sure they get enough sleep throughout the day. The reason why I need to get enough sleep is to ensure that your hormones are producing optimally throughout the day. When you're sleeping not only recovering from the rest of the day but you're also boosting your growth hormone and other hormones which are related to health and wellness.

You need to make sure that you get enough sleep throughout the day as we said before 6 to 8 hours is optimal for people looking to get the health benefits from sleeping. When intermittent fasting, in the beginning, you might find it hard to sleep. The reason why is because you adrenaline might be high throughout the day and will continue to stay that high later that night, a couple of ways to ensure they get enough sleep throughout the day while intermittent fasting is by perhaps meditating.

Meditation has shown to help people get into a calm mental state which will help you sleep better. Please do whatever you have to do to get those 6 8 hours of sleep, as it is very crucial for your health and overall success following intermittent fasting.

Autopay

You might have heard claims such as intermittent fasting having anti-aging properties, and there is some truth behind it. When you are following an eating protocol related to fasting your body will start a process known as autophagy. Autophagy is a process when your cells essentially eat themselves and produce newer and stronger ones this process is known as autophagy. When you are eating regularly, your body has to work hard on digesting the foods which you are consuming and then doesn't have the time or energy to activate autophagy.

Which is why you will see amazing results when intermittent fasting because when you are fasting, you are not digesting any food hence having more time for your body to activate the process of rejuvenating new cells. For you to see amazing results from autophagy, you will have to fast for at least 12 to 16 hours. The reason being is that your body will have burned out all the glycogen in your liver to get the process started, another thing to remember is to not fast for two days at a time, as this is when autophagy slowly drops. Overall if your goal is to live longer, you need to have an autophagy process running in a healthy manner which fasting provides you.

Other tips

Now to close out this chapter, let's talk about a couple of things you need to consider when following intermittent fasting or some tips that might help you while observing intermittent fasting. The main thing that will help you when observing intermittent fasting is to make sure that everything is on point.

Make sure though you diet it's okay, your sleep is in check and your exercising in check. When everything is in check, you will see the results that you are looking for. Another tip we would like to give you is to make sure that you ease into intermittent fasting. If you don't ease into it, chances are you might quit, and once you stopped, then there are lot fewer chances of you trying it again. Just start slowly, and increase your fast from there really feel of intermittent fasting before you start messing around with longer fasts. Before you start any of those, make sure you consult your physician or doctor to see if you're healthy enough to follow intermittent fasting.

Chapter 6: How to Start a Diet

By now you should know many things which are related to intermittent fasting, so let's talk about the steps you need to take before you start your intermittent fasting diet.

Before You Get Started

Before you get started, there are a couple of things to understand about intermittent fasting. The first thing is going to be making sure that intermittent fasting is followed the right way, as described in this book. If you don't do it right then chances of you achieving your goals will go down significantly, so make sure you read this book very carefully before you start any fat intermittent fasting diet protocol.

Consult a Health Physician

Before you start any diet, you need to consult with your position. As we talked about before how intermittent fasting cannot be suited for some people out there oh, so it is in your best interest to figure out if you are well enough to follow intermittent fasting. Ideally, you want to consult with someone, whom you can trust perhaps your doctor or a dietitian. However, whatever you do you make sure that you consult with a professional who knows what they're doing since we don't see what you look like or what your health complications are we can tell you if you're fit enough for intermittent fasting or not. If you aren't fit enough for intermittent fasting, then perhaps try something new.

Keep It Easy

Keeping it easy one of the best things you can do to your body Because the truth is it needs to feel less like a chore and more like a lifestyle so if you want to be successful in this, then it needs to feel comfortable. If you feel like intermittent fasting is a chore for you from the get-go, then the chances of you continuing with intermittent fasting will go down drastically. Whatever you do, make sure the intermittent fasting feels comfortable for you and that it is not a chore but more so of a lifestyle.

Now there's a couple of ways to keep it easy, and the first way would be to start slow. We have to explain to you how to start easy, so start with that and then move on to the big stuff. Overall you want to make intermittent fasting and easy manageable part of your life, and you have to figure out how you're going to do that. We can give you some pointers and some tricks on how to do that, but it is for you to find out what works for you and what doesn't.

Keep It Simple

Please don't make things harder than they're supposed to be, especially when you're intermittent fasting. It is straightforward to make things hard when following intermittent fasting, as there many things to consider and many things to do. The best thing you can do is keep things simple; the way to keep things simple is by not overthinking stuff. By that I mean, not overthinking how much food you're missing while fasting or what kind of foods you will be eating when you break your fast. Just take it one step at a time, when you start taking one step at a time is a lot easier for you to continue with intermittent fasting and it won't feel like such a chore.

Also when you try to keep things simple, you need to realize that it is in your best interest to stay away from external information which might throw you off. Such as new diet fads that are coming out, make sure you stay in your lane and follow intermittent fasting for the time being. Please stick to the plan, do not deviate from it and finally keep things simple.

"When should you start intermittent fasting?"

Now we come on to the main question, "When should you start intermittent fasting?" The simple answer to that is whatever time feels right to you. Here's the thing, whatever time fits your schedule and all your needs will work the best, the truth is that intermittent fasting doesn't have a specific time when you fast and when you don't fast. If you're following a 16 hour fast, then you can quickly start your fast at 8 p.m. and break it at 12 p.m. the next day, or whatever time works for you.

Just make sure, that you're fast ends closer to your work out time. Especially for someone looking to put on muscle, make sure whenever you work out you are breaking your fast right after it. This will ensure that you get enough protein in your system to build a muscle back which you broke down, this isn't necessary, but it is an ideal situation. Figure out when you work out, and map out the times he will be fasting and the times you will be eating, and you have your fasting protocol.

Choose Which Days to Fast

Depending on the type of intermittent fasting you're going to be falling, we need to pick out what days you will be fasting what Daisy will not be fasting. Ideally, you want to pick a day when you're doing a lot less work to fast, and when you have more stuff at hand, you can decide to not fast on that day.

Just make sure whatever day you pick, that it is comfortable for you to fast then it is on other days. Like I said before there are no restrictions on the time or the date when you're fasting or non-fasting. As long as you get the things done, you're fasting endeavors would be a good and overall help you achieve your goal.

Forgive Your Slip-Ups

There will be many times that you will be slipping up, but don't worry that happens to everyone. Here's the thing following a routine and sticking to it as a good thing, but we are humans, and we will slip up time, and time again it makes you feel any better I have as well. So when you're fasting, don't think of you slip up those failures feel of it as a stepping stone. Maybe your body needs a break, which is why you had that stuff up.

Moreover, once you do have your slip-ups forgive yourself and move on and start over again. Eventually, you will get to the point that it becomes more for lifestyle, and you won't have any slip-ups anymore. Just keep going at it, don't give up and you will be fine.

"What is your purpose?"

Many people when they're starting intermittent fasting, they figure out the meaning. The truth is that you need to find out why you're following intermittent fasting and what your goals are. So if your goal is to lose weight they need to make sure that that is your only call, and then once you figure out what your goal is you need to pick a plan which works the best for you.

In the later chapters we will show you how to pick a plan out for your goals, just realize that you will still notice many health benefits from all the intermittent fasting, but you got to recognize on some intermittent fasting Protocols are better suited for people who are looking to lose weight rather than see some health benefits.

"What are your concerns?"

You have to forget all your worries when following intermittent fasting, and going to it stress-free. If you have any questions or concerns regarding intermittent fasting, find out what they are and figure them out at how you are going to fix it. Most of the things regarding intermittent fasting will be covered in this book. However, you need to do your research and find out what works for you and what doesn't.

Take Precautions

As we mentioned to you before, you need to take precautions when you're falling intermittent fasting. You need to realize when you're not feeling well when intermittent fasting, which means you need to understand your body.

If you ever feel like you in spite of fasting is causing you more harm and fewer benefits than in his stop intermittent fasting done in there. If you consult with the doctor, then you will know precisely if intermittent fasting is the answer for you or not. Just make sure whatever you were doing, is healthy for you. Taking precautions include many things, but more specifically you are prepared for what is coming when intermittent fasting.

Pregnancy

If you're pregnant, then you should not follow intermittent fasting. The reason why I should not have intermittent fasting is that your body needs regular food all the time to feed you and your infant, so if you are pregnant, then you should not follow intermittent fasting as it is not only in healthy for you, but it will be unhealthy for a child as well.

The chances of you giving up when intermittent fasting while pregnant will be extremely high, the simple reason why is because it isn't safe for pregnant women.

Diabetes

One of the great benefits for intermittent fasting is that it reduces the risk of many diseases, more specifically reduces the risk of diabetes. However, if you already have diabetes, then you should not be falling intermittent fasting here's why.

When you are diabetic you're taking something called insulin. When you are taking insulin, you need regular food throughout the day or else you will go into a glycemic coma.

Once you go into a glycemic coma, chances of surviving would be slim to none.

Believe it or not when intermittent fasting when you're on a diabetic prescription it could be very deadly. So if you have diabetes are facing any health issues for the small consult with the doctor, and sing of all make sure you novel intermittent fasting as it can be deadly.

Electrolyte Imbalance

When you're falling intermittent fasting, the chances of you noticing electrolyte imbalances will be very high. You need to make sure they getting enough electrolytes throughout the day to make sure that your body is functioning correctly. Sometimes, people drink electrolyte drinks while following intermittent fasting, which we don't recommend since I can break your fast.

However, when you do break your fast to get how some electrolyte drinks to replenish electrolytes. Some of the ways to tell the electrolytes are low is to see how you feel throughout the day if you were noticing joint pains lower energy than trans are electrolytes are a little bit on the lower side to make sure that you get that checked. Overall, make sure that once you do break your fast to get all the electrolytes that you need.

Chapter 7: Intermittent Fasting and Ketogenic Diet

The Ketogenic Diet Breakdown

Remember how in the early chapters we told you one diet which will go well with intermittent fasting, now we're going to talk about it. The ketogenic diet is one of the best foods you can follow when intermittent fasting, and there's a reason why. When you follow the ketogenic diet, you are using fat for fuel instead of carbohydrates for fuel.

What this will allow you to do is burn more calories throughout the day, the same thing with intermittent fasting. When you're intermittent fasting, you're burning fat for fuel instead of glycogen for fuel, which is why most people suggest ketogenic diet, when following intermittent fasting. Now there are a couple of things to consider when following intermittent fasting and ketogenic diet together. In the beginning, it will feel tough for you to follow a ketogenic diet and intermittent fasting along, which is why we recognize slowly add ketogenic diet to your fasting protocol once you get used to intermittent fasting.

The way ketogenic diet works is straightforward when you're following the ketogenic diet, you're not eating any carbs, and you're only eating high-fat moderate protein. When you eat high-fat moderate protein, eventually your body goes into something called the ketosis. How to get into the ketosis your body with only use energy from fats instead of glycogen Which is why it goes well with intermittent fasting, that's the will help you burn more calories throughout the day, more specifically burn more fat throughout the day when you follow ketogenic diet together. When you follow the ketogenic diet you make your body produce more ketones, what ketones do is allow your body to use fat for energy instead of anything else. In the next section, we will talk more about ketones and how they work.

More About Ketones

For people that don't know what ketones are, ketones are water-soluble molecules which are produced by the liver and fatty acids. When you're not eating enough food, which includes carbohydrates, your body will go into starvation mode, and once it goes into the starvation mode, it will start using your ketones for energy.

When you have higher levels of ketones in your body will start using any stores available in your body to convert it into energy there are many ways to check if you're producing enough ketones. There's one year until she can get from any drug store, and it will show you if you're producing enough ketones or not. Just remember that for you to be in the ketogenic diet you need to be producing enough ketones and be in ketosis.

Moreover, once you're in ketosis, you will start using fat for energy instead of glycogen for energy. When you mix that up with intermittent fasting, you have a recipe for success to lose body fat. Here's the thing when you're falling intermittent fasting you are increasing your ketones in your body. Moreover, when you add ketogenic diet to the equation, you're further enhancing your chances are boosting ketones in your body. There's nothing else to know about ketones, other than to find out what they do to your body.

How Intermittent Fasting Works

In the earlier days, our ancestors wouldn't have an ample supply of food. Unfortunately, they didn't have a grocery store to go to if they wanted food. The only way they would get fed is by hunting and finding foods, resulting in extended amounts of time without food. However, once they had food, they would make sure to eat as much as possible, so they utilize everything. What would happen is that the body would store the food as fat, and use it for energy for the time they are without food.

Fast forward to present time, where food is readily available to us. We eat at least three to five times a day, making our body use the menu for energy source and not the stored fat. You see, our collection is brilliant at understanding our eating pattern. It will save our fat stores for the rainy days, and use the glycogen found in our diet readily. What intermittent fasting does is trick our body, it makes our body think that we are in a "starvation zone," and we need to use our fat for energy to survive as we did back in the day.

When you break your fast after 16 hours or whichever period, your body will absorb all the food you are eating to feed the brain, organs, and muscles, making it a lot less likely for you to store it into fat. That is mainly because of insulin, and when you are fasting, you tend to become a lot more insulin sensitive. In layman terms, the more sensitive you are to insulin the more likely you will use the energy from food instead of storing it. These changes in insulin will result in lower body fat levels and stronger bones and muscles, making it very good for overall health and wellness.

Eating less frequently will also give your body more time to get rid of any bad stuff in your intestine or body since you are not eating for a prolonged period. Hence, detoxing your body and making it healthier. There are numerous benefits to intermittent fasting, and we will discuss those later in this book. Once you start following intermittent fasting, you will realize that every time you break your fast you won't feel like eating much, your body will make you eat less as it wants to process it more effectively.

Making sure that you absorb the food for its right use, which is to feed the muscles and not store it into fat. Intermittent fasting takes your body into a healthy "starvation mode." Then it uses your fat stores for energy, and once you end up breaking your fast, it will use up all the food in the right way. Hopefully, this taught you many things about fasting now we will move on to the topic of why someone should follow it.

Intermittent Fasting and Ketogenic Diet

As you know when you follow intermittent fasting, you are burning a lot more calories, and therefore it will allow you to burn fat. When you combine a ketogenic diet with intermittent fasting, you will be burning more fat since you don't have to burn any glycogen stores in your bloodstream.

Which is why intermittent fasting is one of the best ways to go about burning fat, and once you add ketogenic diet into conjunction there is no stopping. There are a couple of things to consider when you are picking out the right method of ketogenic diet protocols, one of the things you need to make sure is the ability to eat food during your eating window. You have to remember that you are still following intermittent fasting, meaning you can't mess that up.

As we have said before, you need to ease into the diet and make sure that you are losing weight at a reasonable rate without noticing any other side effects related to intermittent fasting and keto. One thing you might see when following a ketogenic diet is something called a keto flu. This might happen because you are ready for it, so make sure that if you do notice symptoms such as vomiting or lack of strength in the gym. Then you need to consult with your doctor, as we said previously consult with your doctor before you start any diet or nutrition plan.

Chapter 8: Types of Intermittent Fasting

Intermittent fasting has been in use since the early days, people use to fast for two to three days at a time just because they couldn't find food. This method was not used for "losing weight" or to "gain energy" or any other health benefits that fasting can be associated with these days. Fasting was simply a common practice most of the human race did as the food was not as easily accessible as it is now. In the present life where we live, food is something that is really accessible to most of us nowadays as there is a restaurant or a grocery store five minutes away from us. We don't have to wait two-three days to find food as our ancestors did. This drastic change in our lifestyles made us change our eating habits by making us eat more often, and in large quantities. Which some would say has caused us to create diseases like obesity, diabetes, heart diseases and much more.

Does this mean having food available to us 24/7 a bad thing? Does that mean our ancestors were better off when it comes to being physically healthy even though they were underfed for days? There are a lot of things fasting has shown to improve our health and wellness, but that doesn't mean you should be fasting. There are a lot of other ways to improve your health and wellness, but for some, fasting might be the answer to better health and wellness and the only way to find out is to fast for yourself.

A lot of my acquaintances and I have followed a strict fasting protocol and have seen tremendous results from it, Some people say it is the best thing that has ever happened to them, others say it's not worth their efforts. What this book will do for you is list out seven different things on what are the benefits and why you should be fasting. If you are overweight, have high blood pressure, or simply don't have time to eat every 2-3 hours, then fasting might be the answer for your better health and wellness, and this book will be your first step to it. There are tremendous benefits to fasting as fasting should be done by everyone to find out for themselves how it can change their health. So get ready to learn a lot of things that you didn't know about fasting and why those things will help you live a fantastic life when it comes to physical and mental health.

Skipping Meals

This method is something people use to get their body use to fasting, now to be clear I don't consider this to be as beneficial as most fasting protocol, and I repeat I don't believe this method to be as helpful as most fasting protocol. Now saying that would I recommend this method to someone else? The answer is yes! Why you ask, the simple reason this method is one of the easiest to follow, and it prepares you for fasting ways that will help you with physical health and wellness. That being said would I recommend someone make this method their lifestyle no, only consider this if you have never followed a fasting method before and you want to slowly build up to a longer fast then this method is the right one for you. Some readers can completely ignore this method and start with other fasting method's listed in the following chapters, if you have experience fasting before for fifteen days then you should be able to follow a more "intense" method. That being said lets us talk about these "How-To" methods

The whole point of this method is for you to start skipping meals in between the day to ease you into a longer fast. So what you can do if you decide to follow this plan is to start by skipping breakfast then have some lunch and dinner, slowly building up to a longer fast. If you want you can even have a snack instead of skipping breakfast which will make it easier for you. The whole point is to make you feel comfortable before taking the big step, and this method allows you to take baby steps into the vast realm of fasting. Which I think is the plus of this fasting method.

There are some benefits to this type of fasting method. One of the things that you might notice especially starting is that you will most likely lose some fat. Often we don't realize how much we overeat, and an average person tends to eat more than he or she should since most North American diet consists of food that is filled with carbohydrates, sugar and a ton of "bad fat" such as trans-fat in their diet, which leads to most of the obesity issues in our society. One meal on average tends to be six hundred to a thousand calories per meal. Now if you skip one meal every day for a week, you are looking to cut about forty two-hundred to seven thousand calories a week, a pound of fat has thirty five-hundred calories so you can defiantly see some fat loss benefits. This method will also give your gut a break from digesting all this processed food that some readers might be eating, which means better gut health overall.

You can see all the benefits of this method, but this fasting method is something that you should not use as a protocol to lose fat in the long term as it can leave you malnourished in the end. See my primary goal with this book is to show you how to live a healthy life both physically and mentally, sometimes our body gives us signals to skip meals and without even knowing you would skip a meal just because you felt like it. So we are Always using this method anyways, but then the next day instead of three we have four meals and not to mention a big and unhealthy one. So our body always makes us clean our gut time to time organically, one thing people can get carried away within this method is since they skip a meal they think they can have anything their heart desires. Which should not be the case, in my opinion, you need to be eating healthy doesn't matter if you choose to fast or not if you want to be free of health complications in future to looking and feeling good. By eating healthy we make sure to get all our micronutrients in, like our vitamins and minerals for the day and your macronutrients like your calories, fats, carbs and protein depending on your fitness and aesthetic goals. Another thing that should not be left out is the consumption of water if you can't seem to skip the meal and you tend to get hungry, drink more water during your fast. Not only will that hydrate you, but it will also get rid of toxins in your body and help you with fat loss if that's your goal. At the end of the day, if you want to ease into this fasting lifestyle, you should use this method as a tool to get you up to a longer fast so you don't fall off track as you could have if you started with a more extended method for fasting.

The "Basic" Fasting Method

The method which we will be discussing in this chapter will be the most commonly practiced method in fasting, and this method involves fasting for fourteen to sixteen hours and having an eating window of ten to eight hours depending on how long you decide to fast. The method is known as the "16/8" method, as most of the people choose to fast for sixteen hours instead of fourteen hours hence the name. The whole point of this method is that all the fasting is based on hours. Meaning that instead of fasting for days you fast every day for the specified amount of hours, this method, in my opinion, is the most convenient method to follow as this is also the methods that helped me get down to the lowest body fat percentage.

Commonly used by people who want to look more aesthetically pleasing, this method has less risk of you losing your muscle mass while still losing body-fat. Especially for people who follow a strict workout regimen, this fasting method would be optimal for you as you don't have to be fasting the whole day, which means you get nutrients in your body every day. Those nutrients can be used to repair torn muscle fibers quicker than most fasting methods. Also, this method is the easiest one to follow in my opinion and others I know who have followed a fasting lifestyle.

The whole point of this fasting phase is to fast for certain hours of the day and eat for specific hours of the day. I would highly recommend you start by fasting for fourteen hours and have an eating window of ten hours to eat. After you feel comfortable following "14/10" method slowly increase it to the "16/8" fasting method, this will ensure you don't go "crazy "and break the fast-starting off since you will be easing into it. Now some sources are saying that women should only fast for fourteen to fifteen hours as they seem to do better on them, I would recommend you build up to fasting for sixteen hours and see how you like it before you think about scaling down.

When following this method, you are allowed to have no calorie drinks so water, black coffee and other calorie-free drinks that you might like. One thing I would not recommend having while fasting is branched-chain amino acids intake, which mostly used by bodybuilders and fitness enthusiasts to preserve their muscles during workouts and between meals. The reason is it will break your fast since it has three amino acids in them known as leucine, isoleucine, and valine, which are indeed macronutrients and will break down in your body in the same manner as protein would. One gram of branched-chain amino acid tends to have six calories, so now you can see how this can break your fast.

This method is the most basic and also useful for seeing the physical changes and health benefits that you will be seeing from fasting anyways. However, keep in mind to eat healthy foods in your eating window, fasting doesn't mean you can have anything you want and look at the results. This method would be great for someone whose lifestyle does not allow him to have food often throughout the day. This will make it easy for you to follow a healthy lifestyle without affecting other things in life. Make sure to start with a shorter fasting period than sixteen hours, slowly build up to fasting for sixteen hours. All in all this method is basic easy to follow, and it works great, and you will defiantly get out of this method what you're looking for which is looking great and being healthy.

How to exactly go about following this fasting protocol is simple, and you can do it in two ways. The first protocol would be skipping breakfast and starting your day off with your first meal at 12 pm and keep hitting your macronutrient needs for the day till 8 pm. This is the preferred method by most people as you get to eat at the prime times of the day when you would be hungry anyway. Also, it makes it easier for you to get a workout in a while keeping your body supplied with an ample amount of protein for the right amount of time. Not that fasting will make you lose your muscle's, but it sure gives most people a peace of mind, The next protocol would be to have your breakfast at 8 am and keep feeding yourself till 4 pm. This tends to get a bit tough mentally in the beginning stages of fasting as you don't get to eat anything after 4 pm, most of you guys still have a chunk of your day left, follow this if it suits your daily lifestyle better. Best way to go about this method is to find your optimal hours to fast and the optimal hours to feed, and one tip would be not to have your feeding window when you are supposed to be sleeping as you don't want to lose your sleep over-eating.

The Warrior Diet

This method is more based on our ancestors' eating habits. Created by Ori Hofmekler, this method suggests us to "eat like a warrior." In the earlier times by fasting thru out the day and only having a four-hour window of having a big meal, as Hofmekler thinks human were created to eat like this. This method was based on his belief system and how humans should be eating instead of using science-based evidence and studies. In this method, you are allowed to mostly have whatever you want in that four-hour eating window, go by what you feel and also don't go by macronutrient count eat how much ever you want to eat.

Another thing that is advocated in this method is that you will be more suited for burning fat for energy, claimed by Ori Hofmekler. If you follow this diet, you will get lean and won't have to count calories to lose body fat. So in this method, you have you fast for twenty hours and have an eating window of only four hours. Now if you are currently using the "16/8" method then switching up to the warrior diet won't be such a shock to your body but if you are going to go from an average eating habit to this, then I will be hard for you physically. I would recommend starting with fasting for fourteen hours and slowly building up to the twenty-hour mark. If fasting for fourteen hours can get challenging for you, then I would suggest slowly skipping meals like breakfast and then when that feels easy slowly skipping breakfast and lunch, till you get to the point where you can fast for twenty hours of the day.

Now, the way its recommend to follow this method is to fast in the day time and eat at the night time, as warriors would after hunting and preparing their meals at the end of the day. You can have your meals at any time even before going to bed, and this diet should be followed just like the ancient times like the warrior did, meaning fast in the morning and feast at night. In this diet, you can have fruits and vegetables but its recommended you stay away from canned fruits and vegetables, also their juices.

In this method, it's highly recommended to workout in an empty stomach, I am guessing to stimulate a warrior lifestyle. It is suggested to exercise for thirty to forty-five minutes of intense workouts, with the use of compound movements like pull-ups, push-ups, and squats which use more than one muscle group. You can still consume water, and other no-calorie drinks so don't be scared to workout not hydrated.

In conclusion, this diet is based on a lifestyle that warriors had back in ancient times, which is a selling factor to some people including me. Since this diet has no science or studies to back it up, it can be a turn off to some people when it comes to following a fasting protocol since they might want to see health benefits like lowering the risk of diabetes and other things of that nature. Even though this method is quite similar to "16/8" and I think it should help lower risk of diseases but then again no research on it, but on the other hand, if your goal is to feel and look like a warrior, this method will be the right one for you. Although I haven't followed this plan long enough to see drastic physical changes, I have met people who have completely transformed their physical appearance and health also their energy levels have drastically changed for the better. This method has resulted in success for most people, and when I followed it for one week, I felt like "16-8" is ideal for me as I was seeing and feeling the same on this method. One thing I didn't like about this method is that you have to work out on an empty stomach, with "16/8" I would workout fed. So if you don't mind working out on an empty stomach and you want to live a warrior lifestyle, then this method might be for you.

Even though this goes with no saying, always get recommended by your doctor before you follow this method or another method listed in this book. This method can be pretty hard for you, in the beginning, make sure you don't go into it without easing yourself into the method. I hope you see the results that you are looking for following this fasting method if you chose to pick this method.

Alternate Day Fasting

One of the ways you can start fasting is by using a method called alternate day fasting. Known as one of the best practices to see a decreased risk of chronic diseases like diabetes, cardiovascular diseases, and many others, in human studies, it has shown to bring up "good cholesterol" which led to lower risk of heart diseases. In animals using this method has proved to lower cancerous cells, so without a doubt, this fasting method will be ideal for you if your goals are to prevent the risk of having these diseases. Just like most other fasting methods, it will also help you with goals like fat-loss and other aesthetic purposes that you might have, but this method is more known to lower risk of diseases and used by people who have that goal in mind. This method can still be used with success if you have the goal of losing weight and looking good. Just like others have used this method to lose body fat or put on muscle. That being said let us talk about how this method is to be used.

Well, the name says it all, you will be fasting for one day and then eating a regular healthy diet like you should be the next day. Now on your fasting day, you are not going to be completely restraining yourself from food, you should still have one-fourth of the calories that you have on the non-fasting day. So if you have two thousand calories a day then on fasting days you should be consuming five hundred calories a day on your fasting days, now I would recommend having one meal on your fasting day which should cover your daily requirement for approximately five hundred calories. Some people have also seen some great success with having small snacks throughout the day to equal their calorie need for the day, but that's something I would not recommend you do, but to each their own. That being said let us dive into the pros and con of this method.

There are many pros to this type of method, one of which we already talked about is that it lowers the risk of diabetes. Studies are showing that using this method has decreased the risk of diseases like Diabetes, Cardiovascular diseases, and Cancer so in my eyes this would be an excellent idea for you to start following if your goal is to live a generally healthy life. That being said, to see benefits you will have to eat a clean, healthy diet, just because you are fasting doesn't mean you can eat whatever your heart desires as this mistake is made often by followers of this method.

Another benefit of this method is it will help you lose body fat if that's your goal, there are also different studies showing that using this method over traditional methods helps you lose more body fat compared to conventional methods. Readers who are in the obese side will see some great results from this method when it comes to weight loss. Another benefit of this method could be that it will be easier to follow for weight loss over the traditional methods since conventional methods require you to eat in a pretty substantial caloric deficit whereas in this method you have a lot more wiggle room to eat what you want on your non-fasting days. Like I have stated before, you still have to eat healthy to see results but compared to a traditional diet you can have a lot more foods that are higher in fats and carbs, in moderation of course, please don't eat pizza every non-fasting day and expect to see some great results. That being said don't be shy to have good tasty meals which are also healthy, no need to have bland and unfilling foods like you would in a traditional diet. That being said let's talk about some issues you can face following this method

Although this method might have a lot of benefits, there are some drawbacks to this method. The main one is that it can affect your workouts on fasting days if you are the type of person who likes to exercise, this method could affect your strength negatively. One way to fix this issue is by working out first thing the morning on an empty stomach when its fasting day and then having a meal after the workout, or skip your workout all together on the fasting days. Another issue this method can have is that I can be hard to commit in the long term, even though it might be easier to follow in the beginning compared to traditional diet. Since you mainly eat nothing every other day it can get hard, what if you have a birthday party to attend to on your fasting day or any other event does that mean you won't have a good time and have a meal with your friends and family, most likely you will. As you can tell these can be some significant issues for some followers of this method, one way to go about it is to follow this method for six to eight weeks and then move on to another fasting method.

As you can see, this method is one of the better methods to use for all the benefits you are looking for from following a fasting lifestyle. If you think you can fit this method into your lifestyle, then I would suggest you do so because the benefits out weight the cons this method could potentially have. I would highly recommend you try it for yourself for some time and you can fit it in your lifestyle, and you are enjoying this method while seeing the benefit then keep going, this method will surely help you live a healthier life with the body you want.

Eat-Stop-Eat

This method was created by Brad Pilon, who is a fitness expert and was popularized a couple of years ago. This method is more based on the timing of the meals rather than restricting what types of foods you are allowed to eat, which is good if you still want to eat some tasty foods. Studies are showing that brief fasting can help with losing body fat while keeping your muscles better than traditional dieting would, and also just like any other fasting method would in this method you should notice a lower chance of you getting chronic diseases. People in the fitness industry have used this method. Let me tell you they have gone on to see some tremendous physical difference whether it is losing body fat or having a more ripped looking physique, So how does this method work correctly.

The eat-stop-eat title says it all, and it is where you eat for a couple of days eating a reasonable amount of calories and then you completely fast for a day only allowed to have things like black coffee, calorie-free drinks, and water. Your goal is to fast only one to two times a week but its fasting completely, meaning no food for twenty-four hours. However, the creator of this method has stated that you can fast for a mere twenty hours and still see the benefits. Now, I would recommend not to start by fasting twenty to twenty-four hours, perhaps start by fasting only fourteen to sixteen hours for a day and on your non-workout days to if you have a workout plan that you are currently following. By fasting for even one day, Brad Pilon has stated that you will be in a ten percent calorie deficit, which is excellent for weight loss. One of the ways I would set up myself for the whole week is to not fast for two days and fasting the on the third day, so if you start on Monday, I will fast on Wednesday and Saturday if you have decided to fast twice a week. I would start with only one fasting day, and I would keep it on a day when you are not working out or going to work, maybe for you that day could be a Saturday.

On your fasting day, your goal should be to not eat anything for twenty to twenty-four hours, keeping it to only no-calorie drinks and water, on your fasting day you can decide to have what your heart desires in moderation as overeating could hinder fat loss goals. You can still have right about of carbs fats and protein since under eating can also not be beneficial for you in this method. The creator of this method also recommends you engage in resistance training while you are on this method which will help you put on and preserve your muscle while you lose body fat, but try a not workout on fasting days.

There are many benefits to this method, so let us talk about them. One of the benefits is that from personal experiences and others this method will help you lose a lot of body fat without restricting your calories too much, which is excellent since you can melt off a lot of your body fat and still lose weight. Since you are not eating for one to two days a week, this causes you to get into a natural calorie deficit of ten to twenty percent for the week which is what you want if you want to lose body fat. Another great benefit of this diet is that it will help you clean out all the harmful bacteria in your gut since you won't be eating for one to two days a week you will be cleaning out your stomach which will help you digest food better, feel better and look better. This is a significant benefit, as most of you know to have good gut health not only helps with fat loss and mental well-being it also helps you reduce the risk of diseases. As you can see there are many benefits to this diet, now let us talk about some problems that you can have with this method.

One of the major flaws is that this method won't be suitable for some. If your work life is pretty physically demanding well fasting on a weekday can get a bit problematic, since you need some calories to move and get thru your work hours. If you decide to work out that day, then you might be hindering your results from this method by being to physically active on fasting days.

Even though this method is only to be followed for two days, you can have some problems going thru the whole day fasting. For me it caused me to have the feeling of nausea, headaches and I was irritable at the eighteen-hour mark. I had to use a lot of my will power to continue for the remaining hours, so as you can see this diet does require much willpower on your fasting days. I would suggest slowly building up to twenty-four hours so you can get used to fasting and make it easier for yourself.

In conclusion, this method is excellent for fat loss and better gut health. Not only will you lose fat and preserve muscle on this method you will also lower the risk of diseases and have better gut health. I can't stress enough how important it is to have excellent gut health, it is crucial since having a healthy gut means having a healthy body overall. I would highly recommend this method to someone who is looking to get lean while preserving muscle, as this method works best for people who are aiming towards the goal of having a more aesthetically pleasing body and for people who want to refresh and clean your gut this method could be the one for you.

The 5:2 Method

This fasting method was popularized by Michael Mosley, who is a doctor and journalist. Since this method has no studies to prove its benefits, it is still a fasting method, and this fasting has shown some benefits. The benefits that are claimed includes Better brain function, Reducing the risk of heart disease, stroke, cancer and improving cholesterol levels, just like any fasting methods would. This method can get tough to follow for some people, but it will put you in a twenty percent calorie deficit which is where you want to be if your goal is to lose body fat. This could be an excellent way to use this method if you can handle it. On that note, let's talk about this method and how it works.

The 5:2 method is where a person eats an average amount of calories throughout the week and restricts their calories to five hundred to six hundred calories a day for two days. The guideline says five hundred calories a day for women and six hundred calories for men on fasting days. The method recommends on your fasting days you have two meals divided into your calories for the day, meaning two meals of two fifty calories for women and two meals of three hundred calories a day for men. So your calories will be entirely restricted throughout those two days, make sure you are drinking a ton of water and other no-calorie liquids during your fasting days.

Now, the best way that you can go about using this method of fasting would generally be eating thru Monday to Friday then fasting over the weekend, and my recommendation would be fast when you don't have work or if you are doing anything physically demanding like working out. This will ensure you don't feel tired or worst go hypoglycemic as you will be "fasting" for quite a long time, so make sure you are fasting on days you are not working or doing anything physically demanding. Also, the great thing about this method is that there is no food restriction during non-fasting days, which is a good thing for some you foodies out there. Now there are some benefits to these methods, let's talk about that.

The primary benefit is that you will lose body fat and that too quite quickly as you will be eating so little during those two days of fasting. I have personally followed this plan just as an experiment and I have to say, and I did lose body fat in those two weeks that I followed it. If your goal is fat loss without restricting your diet as much, then this method can be the one for you. Another benefit claimed are lower cholesterol, lower risk of heart disease and cancer, which is fantastic for everyone following this method of fasting. However, then again these benefits are claimed, not proven so don't support this method if your goal is to lower the risk of diseases there are other fasting methods in this book that you can follow to get those benefits. The great thing about this fasting method is that you will get to eat what you want to eat, no need to restrict yourself on non-fasting days, but if I were you, I would still be careful not to overeat if your goal is to lose body fat. Those are the benefits, now let us talk about the cons.

This method is not perfect by any means, there are some flaws to this method, and one of them was used in a positive way but is also used as a con. In this method, you can eat whatever you want to eat, which is a flaw since people will eat a lot of junk food as an excuse and not do any justice to their health. I believe that fasting should be accompanied with a well-balanced, healthy diet and not having junk food here and there. I would not say I like the fact of having whatever you want on your non-fasting days as it can take away from the benefits of fasting.

Another flaw of this method is that it can be tough for some people to make it a lifestyle as fasting for two days straight can be a problem, but if it works for you then go for it. The main flaw is that there is no backing up the claims that this method has made. Although this is a fasting method and fasting has many benefits that have been backed up, this method doesn't so as I said before don't follow this diet if your sole purpose is to lower the risk of diseases. If you develop a workout plan that requires strength training what you should be doing for a healthier life and body, then this method can hinder your workout quality as for some people it did.

Now you know all about the 5:2 method, this method can be used with great success if your goal is to lose body fat and have no restrictions to your diet on non-fasting days. However, please use this method for the right reasons, don't use it if you want a lowered risk of diseases as studies have not proved it. Other fasting methods can be followed if your goal is lower the chances, and if your goal is to get stronger and put on some muscle then this method won't be ideal as this method can affect your workouts. All in all this method used for the right reasons then it can be used with great success.

The Water Fast

Well, the name says it all this method has got to be one most laborious fasting methods that you can follow. Most of the ways can be used for an extended period, but I would suggest this method is only used only certain times a year. I would use this method as a tool, rather than a lifestyle as doing this for too long can do some damage to your body. That being said this method can be used to your advantage, but first, let's talk about how this method works.

This method is based on you eating like you normally would, and then fasting for one to three days with the only thing that you can have during your fasting period is water. The best way to start this fast is to plan it ahead of time, slowly lower the calories every day as you get closer to your water fast as it will prepare your body and it won't be such a shock. An example will be if you were consuming two thousand calories day what I would recommend is to lower five hundred calories every day so on the fourth day you can start your fast without it being a shock. Now the best way to go about fasting is to fast for one to two days no longer than three days, some people have fasted for ten days using this method, but I would not recommend you go without food for that long, and I don't see the reason why you should be fasting for so long.

Since there are not many guidelines on how often you should fast using this method, the best way would be to use this method is to fast every four to eight weeks and I wouldn't go past three days of actual fasting. I would recommend you fast on days that you are not doing anything physically like working out since it can affect your workout and your whole day after that. One thing I would recommend you don't do is to use this method more than twelve times in a year, as doing it often can affect in your day-to-day life and energy levels based on experiences. Although this method can't be used as a lifestyle, there are some benefits to these methods, so let us talk about them.

This method is best known for cleaning out toxins in your body. Since you won't be eating for one to three days and the only thing that you will be consuming is water, your body will automatically get rid of toxins in your body with the help of water. This has got be a selling point for me when it comes to using this method, don't get me wrong every fasting method helps with cleaning out your body, but if your body doesn't ingest anything for one to three days, then that gives your body plenty of time to "clean up." Another wonderful benefit of using this method is that it will clean out any harmful bacteria in your gut, which will help you digest your food better the next time you consume some. Since you will be getting rid of toxins in your body, you will also get the benefit of lowered risk of diseases which is always a plus.

Another thing this method can help you with is a fat loss since you won't be eating for so long your body will depend on fat for energy, but I would not use this method for fat loss as

There are other methods that you can use for that goal. As you can see this method has some benefit, now let us talk about some issues that you can have with this method.

The first issue with this method is that it can be super hard to go thru with. Fasting for one to three days with no food requires a lot of will power, and often people won't go thru with this method since it's so hard. Another issue that this method could have is that it can affect your strength. If you are into strength training, then be prepared to lose some power following this plan too often. This issue can be kept in control if you fast on non-workout days and use this method every four to eight weeks. One of the major flaws with this method is that there is a chance that you can go hypoglycemic, so be careful as this can get super dangerous if you fast for an extended period. These are the main issues with using this method, most of the problems can be fixed if you be careful and don't use this method often meaning not exceeding more than three days of fasting and easing into the technique.

In conclusion, if used for the right reasons this method can indeed help you with better health by cleaning our body with toxins and improving our gut health. The best way to think about this method is to think about it as a tool instead of a lifestyle, only use this method to clean out your body of all the toxins build up in your body and gut from all the eating that you have been doing for the past one to six months. Give your body a break from digesting and let it clean itself internally. I have to say this is one of the best ways to detoxify your body of harmful Bactria and toxins, which will not only help us digest our food better but also lower the risk of diseases. However, then again down forget to use this as a tool instead of a lifestyle, as it can lead to some dangerous side effects. All in all great for using it to cleanse your body internally which will only make you feel and look better, and lower the risk of diseases.

Overall Benefits that Come with Intermittent Fasting

There are many methods, a time frame which you can follow in intermittent fasting, as we will be discussing multiple types of fasting strategies, about how our ancestors did fasting and they would have to wait for twenty-four to forty-eight hours sometimes even longer before they can find food for themselves. This sure sounds like a tough life and to be honest, it probably was. They were living in a "live or die" type of situation. Although they had a rough life, they still did not have to suffer from diseases like diabetes, high blood pressure, obesity and things of that nature.

I know that most of the ancestors would die at an early age from different reasons, but that doesn't mean we can't learn something from them and use it to our benefits so we can live a healthy better-valued life and mostly not be attracting these human-made diseases. So let us talk about the significant benefits of fasting.

One of the considerable benefits of fasting would be that It helps with fat-loss. Most of the people who are fasting tend to drop body fat percentage especially when they are in a caloric deficit. I have personally achieved my lowest body fat percentage level by using one of the fasting methods. How this works when you are in a fasted state is your insulin levels tend to drop low which means no sugar will be transported from your blood into your fat cells. Instead, you will be using your fat stores for energy most of the time. One advice would be not to work out when you are in your fasting window as your body can start breaking down your muscle for energy instead exercise one or two hours before you break your fast or do your exercises in your feeding window.

A significant benefit of fasting is that it can help with is lowering your risk of diabetes, since your insulin does not keep spiking up while your fasting you become less insulin resistant. Which means your cells won't fail to respond to insulin and your body will be able to use up all the sugar in your blood keeping your blood sugar low. See, when you are diabetic, you are insulin resistant; sometimes, you have to take synthetic insulin as your body doesn't produce the hormone efficiently.

Another thing of having high levels of blood sugar is that it can have an effect on your blood pressure, it can cause you to have high blood pressure if your blood sugar is high. So fasting can help you reduce the risk of diabetes and high blood pressure. In some fasting methods you are allowed to have no to low-calorie drinks like black coffee, don't be surprised your blood pressure goes up after drinking coffee it has nothing to do with insulin and blood sugar, it is a temporary effect when your blood pressure goes up with coffee. So don't confuse the two if you decide to get your blood pressure checked after some time of fasting and you had just consumed some coffee.

Fasting also helps us boost our levels of growth hormone which is responsible for fat loss, muscle gain, and bone density. These things will help us be a healthier person and if your goal is to lose body fat and look muscular then having a higher growth hormone levels is crucial. One of the best things that fasting can help you with is improving your stomach or gut health, so what happens is our good bacteria in your stomach get a break from digesting all the food that we where use to frequently having. Which means our good bacteria can focus on cleaning up our gut even further having fewer toxins in your body and absorbing your food even better.

As you can see there are some fantastic benefits from following a fasting protocol, there are a lot more benefits to fasting, but these are the main ones for our general population. I hope these benefits have convinced you to perhaps live a healthier and a better life with the help of fasting. Not only will fasting help you with all the things above, but it will also help you stay consistent since most of our lifestyles cannot allow us to have a meal even two to three hours like advertised in major fat-loss diets. Which makes most of our lives easier, I am sure it will be hard to start this lifestyle but once you do you will start seeing the benefits which will encourage you to keep going. Please don't give up, keep it going, and eventually, you will get used to this lifestyle and see the results that you have been looking for.

Conclusion

First and foremost, thank you so much for downloading the book *"**The Best Intermittent Fasting Diet**: The Complete Beginner's Guide to Intermittent Fasting for Weight Loss, Cure the Weight Problem, and Reverse Chronic Diseases While Enjoying!"*

Thank you so much for taking the time out and reading my book. I really hope this book has helped you in some way or another to live a healthier life. In my opinion, fasting is one of the best ways to live your nutritional lifestyle since we have evolved to live like this. Our bodies also need a break from eating all of this food so they can clean themselves internally, which lowers the risk of diseases.

Before you start using methods listed in the book, make sure you consult with your physician before you start using one of these methods. Although this book is an eye-opener for most of you, there is still a lot more pros and cons to fasting that have not been scratched in this book. This book is an unbiased review and information on how to use all the primary methods of fasting, and also the pros and cons of each fasting methods which will help you make a proper decision on which one to follow based on your goal and needs.

That being said, I hope you got what you were looking for in this book, find the right fasting method, and use it to your benefit. Thanks again and have fun seeing great results from fasting!

The Easy Intermittent Fasting for Women

The Complete Beginners Guide for Permanent Weight Loss, Burn Fat in Simple and Heal Your Body Through the Self- Cleansing Process of Autophagy

By:

Susan Johnson

Introduction

Congratulations on downloading "The Easy Intermittent Fasting for Women: The Ultimate Beginners Guide for Permanent Weight Loss, Burn Fat in Simple, Healthy, and Scientific Ways, and Heal Your Body Through the Self-Cleansing Process of Autophagy," and thank you for doing so.

The following chapters will discuss everything you need to know in order to practice intermittent fasting successfully. The book is a practical guide to help you figure out how to practice the intermittent fasting lifestyle.

The chapters in this book are here to answer any questions you may have about intermittent fasting and help you make the transition to being an intermittent faster. Chapter One walks you through what intermittent fasting is and what it is not. Chapter Two gives insights on how the intermittent fasting process works. Chapter Three explains the weight loss process and rudimentary problems standing in the way of you losing weight. Chapter Four is all about the benefits of intermittent fasting on your body.

As for the second half of the book, the various intermittent fasting protocols you can follow are explored in Chapter Five. The subject of Chapter Six is the precautionary steps you need to take when you begin intermittent fasting, and Chapter Seven busts all the myths that you may have heard about intermittent fasting. Lastly, Chapters Eight, Nine, and Ten will help you be successful once you begin intermittent fasting as they give you pieces of advice on how to get the most out of intermittent fasting, the four pillars you must do, and important tips to keep you motivated. As you can see, there is a lot of great info to help you with your intermittent fasting journey!

"The Easy Intermittent Fasting for Women: The Ultimate Beginners Guide for Permanent Weight Loss, Burn Fat in Simple, Healthy, and Scientific Ways, and Heal Your Body Through the Self- Cleansing Process of Autophagy" will show you all the easy ways to incorporate intermittent fasting into your lifestyle. It is my hope that you will consider the benefits of intermittent fasting and do not let the thought of fasting deter you. Intermittent fasting is possible! You can implement intermittent fasting when planning your meals and/or your family's meals and watch the results start rolling in. No matter if you are a college student, single, or have a family, this book is for you. If you are looking for a way to control diabetes or deal with other chronic illnesses, this book is also for you.

Intermittent fasting deals with one of the most important aspects of health - your diet. You will be able to see results rather quickly once you start. There are ways to improve your weight loss results, but it is important to remember that weight loss is not the only health goal that intermittent fasting provides.

Intermittent fasting is easy, simple, and a relatively painless way to lead a healthier lifestyle. Once you understand its basic principles, you can find ways to incorporate the changes within your lifestyle for maximum health gains. With this book, there are no longer any excuses that will hinder you from committing to this lifestyle. Everything you need to begin and sustain intermittent fasting is laid out for you plainly and simply in this book. This book is grateful to be a part of your transformation and commitment to a healthier lifestyle. Thank you for making a commitment to yourself and to the people who care about you. By the time you finish reading, you'll be able to discuss intermittent fasting with ease and conviction as a proud practitioner.

I'll end the introduction with the words of Plato, "I fast for greater physical and mental efficiency." Maybe you are like Plato. Maybe you want to fast for the mental and physical benefits for yourself. Maybe you are trying to be an example for your friends and family. Whatever your reason for fasting is, this book can help you get started today.

There are plenty of books on this subject on the market, thanks again for choosing this one! Every effort was made to ensure it is full of as much useful information as possible. Please enjoy!

Chapter 1: What is Intermittent Fasting?

Why would one be interested in fasting? Why would someone forego their favorite foods in order to get healthier? Why would someone subject them to the pain of experiencing hunger? This chapter will explain everything fasting and show you the advantages fasting can have in your life. Fasting has been important to many cultures all around the world from ancient to modern times. This chapter will give a brief overview of intermittent fasting is and what it isn't. It will also give you three practical steps you can follow in order to start intermittent fasting.

Fasting and starvation are often lumped together, but they are different. When a person starves, they do not have any food to eat, whereas, fasting is the purposeful foregoing of food. Starvation is out of a person's control; fasting is done by a person in control. Lots of people reported mental clarity, lesser digestion issues, weight loss, easier sleeping, and a simpler, cleaner, more convenient way of eating as a few of the benefits of fasting. It is also important to note that intermittent fasting is not just a diet. It is a lifestyle change where you eat specifically during a set period of time, and you go without eating for another set period of time. Depending on the results you want, you can make the window of time when you eat bigger or the window of time when you do not eat bigger.

Fasting is as old as humankind itself. It has long been touted for its health benefits for the body and spiritual wellness. The benefits of fasting are hard-wired into our body as a biological mechanism against sickness. Think about the last time you were very sick. Did you want to eat? Of course not! As a matter of fact, when you ate, you probably wanted to throw up any of the food you ate. Hence, fasting is a biologic way to protect one's body when you are sick. Not only as an automatic biologic response to sickness, when you look into ancient history, but fasting was also a well-known remedy for illnesses. Greek philosophers often considered intermittent fasting as a solution to getting better. Ancient times document how many doctors prescribing fasting as a way to deal with illness. Despite the lack of modern tools, it is absolutely amazing how doctors knew that fasting and its different variations were a sure-fire way to deal with illnesses.

Additionally, fasting is a common solution to increase concentration or devoutness in the spiritual realm. Ezra Taft Benson, an American politician, and religious leader was right on the money when describing the mental and health benefits of intermittent fasting. Lots of religions practice some form of fasting as a way to connect with the Divine. Christians have fasted as a way to clean mental fogginess and realign their spiritual purpose. Muslims fast every year during Ramadan as a form of spiritual cleansing. Others have used fasting to make political statements which shows the power of fasting has on others as a show of solidarity for important issues that one believes in. Some cultures like Italians and other European countries usually have a heavy lunch and light breakfast or dinner, which as a form of intermittent fasting. Italians are often lauded worldwide for their diet with many others trying to emulate it in their day-to-day life. As you can see, fasting has been everywhere and is an important part of the human experience. Some people think that you need a lot of time and a big budget to get started intermittent fasting. The truth is that you don't need any of those things. You just need the determination and willpower to begin. Essentially, you can get started with 3 easy steps.

- **Choose which fasting method you want to follow.** – There are lots of different methods of fasting you can select from. Once you choose which method, stick to it and begin the process. Do not feel obligated to continue a fasting method if you know that your body is responding negatively. You can always select a different method to follow. Attention will be given to the different intermittent fasting methods you can follow later in the book.

- **Calculate your calories and make sure you have a well-balanced diet.** - Create a meal plan. Decide if you want to be vegetarian or vegan for more intense results. Do not underestimate the importance of counting your calories. Taking the time to plan your meals and make sure your calories are not going over your daily caloric count or under by too much will be the difference to being able to intermittent fasting correctly or not. Some people eat too much or too little. Do not be that person who fasts, but is still unhealthy. If you pay special attention to what you eat, this will help you be that much more successful as an intermittent faster.

- **Decide which exercise you want to follow on the days that you are not fasting.** – If you are going to exercise while fasting, make sure that you choose methods that are conducive to your fasting days. Take it easy on the days that you are fasting and go harder on the days that you are not fasting. If you need a little extra boost for the days you work out, try carbohydrate loading which is bulking up your meals with carbohydrates to help you make it through your workout. For longer fasts, do not worry about trying to exercise while fasting.

Before the chapter ends, a word of caution must be given. There are some people who should not fast. Those include people that have a history of eating disorders, pregnant women, breastfeeding women, teenagers, children and those with type 1 diabetes. Those with chronic illness or even cancers should also consult with their doctors before fasting. The rule of thumb is to always consult with any health professional before you begin fasting. While it is great to have the desire to want to do intermittent fasting, before you begin, you will first want to check with your health professional before embarking on the fasting journey no matter if you are healthy or not. This is important to make sure you are fasting healthily and safely.

Intermittent fasting should not make you feel sick. Don't be fooled; you will feel hunger, but if at any point, you begin to feel weird while fasting or run into any issues, keep an open line of communication open with your doctor or preferred health care provider. Now that you have a better understanding of what intermittent fasting is and what it isn't, it's time to go into more detail about how intermittent fasting works.

Chapter 2: How Does Intermittent Fasting Work?

Intermittent fasting is not a miracle cure for losing weight. It is a method of losing weight that focuses on creating new habits. Many people have success with intermittent fasting because it is a lifestyle change. Once they get into the habit, they realize that they do not want to stop. This chapter will explain more about intermittent fasting and why it helps you lose weight. It will clear up misconceptions about calorie intake and weight loss that you may have. By the time you finish reading, you will feel confident in the ability of intermittent fasting to help you lose weight.

Because intermittent fasting allows only a certain amount of time to eat, some people feel that they will gain weight. However, this is not the case at all. The best thing about intermittent fasting is that it fits into your lifestyle. You can choose to decide when to eat your meals. Of course, if you are eating lots of junk food and carbohydrates only, overeating and not eating vegetables or fruit with a late eating window, you may gain weight.

The key to intermittent fasting is moderation and balance. If you are eating a normal portion at night, you should not see weight gain. Again, it depends on your body. Keep notes in your food journal (more on that, later in the book) to see how your body reacts to eating at a later window. If you are operating at a calorie deficit, you should be fine. The most important thing is not to overeat to avoid giving yourself a stomach ache and extra calories.

Another popular misconception people have about intermittent fasting is that they will lose muscle instead of fat over time. When you eat, your body releases the nutrients you need steadily over time. Until you need to replenish nutrients from your next meal. Many people assume that fasting immediately causes muscle loss which is not the case at all. When you fast, remember you are still using the nutrients from your previous meal even if it was 16 to 20 hours ago. So realistically, you will not lose muscle weight just by fasting in a certain limited time window. As you continue to learn about intermittent fasting, you will be surprised that it is actually quite healthy and has lots of benefits.

Most of the misconceptions about intermittent fasting are resolved once you start practicing and see how the positive effect it has on your body. Overall, as long as you are counting your calories, you will be fine. Some people feel that you need a trainer or a fad diet to lose weight, but you are able to take your fat loss into your own hands by learning what foods work best with your body.

Most women need about 2,000 calories a day, and most men need to consume about 2,800 calories a day. To lose a pound a week, a person needs to eat about 500 fewer calories daily. Knowing this info can help you craft your meals with maximum weight loss. If you want to experience more weight loss, consider exercising more with your diet. This will make sure you have a more extreme calorie deficient which will increase your weight loss goals. Additionally, when you do eat, you can practice a vegetarian or vegan-based diet. Incorporating a vegan or vegetarian diet is not hard to do if you plan your meals. If you decide to use one of these dietary restrictions, you may also save some money since meat is often more expensive than having a plant-based diet. This will increase your daily caloric intake which will result in more weight loss. However. Be sure to consult with your doctor first and make your changes gradually. If at any point you feel weird or notice any irregularities. You should stop. It cannot be advised how important it is to reach out to your doctor before you begin to set yourself up for yourself. Intermittent fasting is so powerful because it capitalizes on how our body already works.

Intermittent fasting takes advantage of our body's natural cycle of breaking down energy in our bodies. The way fasting works in the body is simple. Our bodies need the energy to run. When we eat, we receive energy from the foods we eat like beans, vegetables, fruits, and carbohydrates to name a few. Our bodies then take sugar or glucose from the food and keep it stored in the muscles and liver. When our bodies need energy, they release it into our bloodstream so our bodies can use it. Yet, when a person begins to fast, our bodies need to get the energy from a different source. After about eight hours of fasting, our livers use most of the glucose that is in our bodies. Our body then goes into gluconeogenesis, which indicates our body is about to enter fasting mode. When a person's body is in gluconeogenesis, this means that the calories that their body burns increases because if the body doesn't have any energy coming it, it makes its own glucose using your body fat. Once the body runs out of fat to use, it then begins to enter into starvation mode. Starving people are in a severe bodily mode in which their body is essentially eating itself to provide nutrients. This mode takes days and months to reach. It is not something that you can enter easily after a few hours of not eating. Intermittent fasting takes advantage of the gluconeogenesis mode that allows your body to burn more calories. This sweet spot of gluconeogenesis is where the leverage of intermittent fasting lies. This sweet spot does not mean you will lose a ton of weight. Rather, it is more measured. As a reminder, people can fast without a doctor's assistance healthily for at least 3 days by drinking water only. Weight loss should be expected, but not dramatic weight loss. However, there are a few things you should be on the lookout once you begin intermittent fasting.

If you begin to think about extreme hunger to the point that you can't do anything else unless you are thinking about food, then intermittent fasting may not be for you. Intermittent fasting should be easy to do. Yes, at times, you will feel hunger. However, you should not be thinking about food so much that you are not able to function. The truth of the matter once you get used to your fasting window, making it won't be an issue. The only concern you should have is if you can't make it through the intermittent fasting window and you cannot function AT ALL. Another indication that intermittent fasting may not be for you is if you experience extreme weight gain, specifically in your mid-area. Unexpected weight gain, which usually is the opposite effect of intermittent fasting should be cause for concern. If at any point, you notice unexpected weight gain, you should definitely reach out to your doctor.

If you have done your research and prepared yourself for the initial rigors of intermittent fasting, it is a safe and healthy option in which to partake. Since you have this book, you are someone concerned about your health, and that's awesome! I applaud you for taking the first step moving forward to taking care of your health. As you keep reading, you will learn more about intermittent fasting and how to safely do it.

Chapter 3: Weight Loss and the Rudimentary Problems in its Way

While losing weight is everyone's dream, there are some things that we must be aware of before we lose weight. This chapter will highlight some of the problems we must be mindful of as our body begins to lose weight thanks to intermittent fasting. There are times when you can lose weight too easily, or you can gain it do is lie. Your goal with intermittent fasting is to lose weight steadily inconsistently by creating a new habit out of the way you eat. Either extreme can point to an issue, so it's important to watch your weight loss once you begin intermittent fasting.

The easiest way to lose weight is by controlling what you eat. Our body sees fat as simple as an excess and stores the fat in our body. The so-called "love handles" and stomach rolls are just extra calories that our body has stored. Losing weight is possible, and our body uses those fat stores when we create a calorie deficit, either by lowering our calorie intake, exercising or a combination of both. However, we can only change our size, not outshape it. When we lose weight, our fat cells shrink. Fat cells are not a problem. Everyone has fat cells. The issue with fat cells occurs when we have more fat cells than necessary. Our body takes the fat we consume and stores them as triglycerides.

If you are overweight, you are at risk of having higher triglycerides which are an indication of higher cholesterol. Women are already at a higher risk of having higher triglycerides which translates into higher cholesterol levels due to normal changes associated with menopause. However, diet is another way that cholesterol levels can go up. If you are not eating well, intermittent fasting can help you be more mindful about what you eat and can help you lower your cholesterol levels.

Thinking about your health is an important part of the human experience and one that many people should pay more attention to. Unfortunately, Americans do not just have full stomachs with fasting never even entering their minds. They are not even eating healthily or even using moderate portions. Americans are plain ol' overeating, and as a result, Americans are suffering from a health crisis.

Over the years, statistics show that the increase in obesity has trended upward and continues to do so. The Centers For Disease Control and Prevention, also known as the CDC, reports that about 40% of American adults and 19% of American children are obese. Simply put, there are a lot of people suffering from obesity and unhealthy lifestyle choices. How does a wealthy country with access to the latest health technologies, free education, and 24-hour gyms arrive at a point where most of its citizens are obese? Health researchers have also asked this question and come to a few conclusions.

The first reason obesity is an unfortunate American culture is because Americans tend to eat restaurants a lot more than they did in the past. According to the *Bloomberg Report*, in 2015, Americans spent more time and money going out to restaurants rather than buying their own groceries, cooking said groceries and eating a healthy, delicious meal at home. While this statistic by itself is not that startling, the next one is. The CDC reports that restaurant portions are now four times more than they were in the 1950s. Thus, if a person is eating out more, they are also consuming more calories which equate to weight gain since. This disregard for portion size is having an adverse effect on health nationwide, and waistlines are expanding as a result. What's more disturbing is that it has sneakily gone up, and most people are not concerned at all.

Additionally, many are being bombarded with ways to live an unhealthy lifestyle. Advertisers take advantage of all the ways to reach the consumer and just double down on all the ways they can eat and should be eating. The UConn Rudd Center for Food Policy found that in 2014, "food companies spent $1.28 billion to advertise snack foods on television, in magazines, in coupons, and, increasingly, on the internet and mobile devices. Almost 60 percent of that advertising spending promoted sweet and savory snacks, while just 11 percent promoted fruit and nut snacks. And advertising of sweet snacks increased 15 percent, even from 2010 to 2014." No matter where you turn, there are advertisements tempting you to fall into the trap of unhealthy living and many people fall for it by eating out more, snacking on unhealthy, processed foods and not exercising. But what about those who eat at home? Are they not less obese than those who eat out? Unfortunately, not so much. They have their own sets of issues to deal with when trying to eat healthily.

Interestingly enough, healthy food is much more expensive than junk food. If you want to purchase organic, healthy foods, then you are looking at a hefty increase in your food bill. If you do not have money to pay for healthy food, like many Americans, guess what you are going to go for? That's right- less healthy food options. And less healthy food options mean more calories which mean more weight gain, especially if there is not a way to work off the excess calories.

Those with higher education tend to have lesser rates of obesity weights as well as those with higher incomes according to the CDC. In other words, the trends in this country point to healthy eating being a luxury of the highly-educated and rich. They can afford to eat healthy by buying the healthiest foods. Since they have incomes that allow them to have more free time than lower-income people, they can also afford to take the time to work out or pay for a gym membership that could offset any gain in calories that they may consume. Disturbingly, being healthy seems to be a benefit only a few can afford. Unfortunately, trying to live a healthy lifestyle is difficult, and you are going to run into obstacles that will support you being obese. The statistics show that many are falling prey to the obesity epidemic.

Being obese can set one up for a lifetime battle with chronic illnesses. The more obese you are, the higher your chances are of getting chronic diseases like heart disease, diabetes, or stroke. The CDC notes that "Obesity-related conditions include heart disease, stroke, type 2 diabetes and certain types of cancer that are some of the leading causes of preventable, premature death." The saddest part about being obese is that it is totally preventable. A simple diet and mental change can help people with obesity prevent their untimely demise. I do not want you to fall prey to the ills the obesity. Despite their being solutions to handling and dealing with weight concerns, most people have no idea about how to control their diets or even begin the journey to a healthier lifestyle.

There are lots of people who struggle with their weight. They jump back and forth between fad diet after fad diet seeing limited to no results. Some people may go to the gym one week and the weeks do not go at all. They have no motivation or desire to be healthy. Other people are so busy with their families and careers that they do not have time to give attention to their health, especially their diet. These people pick up fast food on the way to work and on the way home, and their bodies are taking a major hit. Other people are interested in being healthy but have no idea where to begin. Everyone knows that you should prioritize your health, but if you have never been talked or seen healthy habits practiced, they run around like a chicken with its head cut off. Feeling discouraged about not knowing where to begin their health (if they even care at all), all of these people just give up and succumb to a lifestyle of unhealthy eating and unhealthy habits. All of us have been one of these people in life. Maybe you are one of these people, who has hit rock bottom, and you know that you have to do something about your health or you will suffer dire consequences. Look no further.

Thankfully, for those who are trying to be healthy, there is light at the end of the tunnel. There is a way for you to get your weight under control and to be the healthy person that you know you can be. This method also works for people who are already healthy as well. The easiest way to get healthy is to gain control of your diet. If you can control your diet, gaining or losing weight becomes a lot easier. Even for those who have had to struggle with their diet, there is the help. The easiest way to get your diet under control is by intermittent fasting. Intermittent fasting is all about limiting the time that you eat, with a focus on eating healthy foods when you do eat.

Ultimately, intermittent fasting helps you maintain healthy portion control and lends itself to an overall improvement in one's health. It helps you fight sugar cravings and unsavory inflammatory illnesses that can hinder one for life. It even helps with cholesterol levels. Ultimately, intermittent fasting activates your metabolism and creates a caloric deficit if you are counting your calories which can help you lose weight. If you combine your intermittent fasting lifestyle with a vegan or vegetarian diet, you can lose even more weight. You can use intermittent fasting how you want to in order to reach the goals that you'd like!

Chapter 4: The Impact of Intermittent Fasting on Your Body

There are a number of effects intermittent fasting can have on your body. The most obvious effect, of course, is weight loss. Losing weight is only one benefit of the intermittent fasting lifestyle. Intermittent fasting has numerous benefits with weight loss only being an extra.

Intermittent fasting has been linked to improving mental health, chronic illness, and heart disease, even helping to prevent certain cancers and seizures. Lifestyle change and extended health benefits are what makes intermittent fasting superior to other diets and methods. The best thing about intermittent fasting is, once you get into the habit of doing it, the health results stay with you for years. You do not have to worry about getting into the horrible cycle of gaining weight and losing weight. Intermittent fasting is a habit that is inherently healthy and easier for one to maintain over long periods of time because it is something that you do every day without having to think about it. You can also mold it to fit the most hectic or most laid-back lifestyles.

There are many reasons that people decide to fast. The main draw for many is the potential to lose weight. Fasting does not just help you lose weight, but it helps you to lose weight in one of the most stubborn places - your stomach. How many of us have struggled with trying to lose those love handles and that muffin top! Never fear, intermittent fasting is the solution that you've been looking for to tackle these spots. Because intermittent fasting inherently restricts your meals to a certain time, you are already lowering your daily caloric intake. When you do that, you end up losing weight.

However, intermittent fasting is more effective because it causes your weight loss hormones to rev up. One of the first hormones that increase while you fast is called the human growth hormone. The human growth hormone helps your body burn more fat and increase muscle gain, which helps lose more weight in the process.

When you are in a fasted state, your body gets energy from your body's fat stores and not the food that you are eating. This, in turn, increases your metabolism rate. So what is your metabolism rate? That is the rate at which you lose calories. You can lose calories by either eating less food or getting your body to use your stored fat, which is what intermittent fasting does. A definite win-win. Additionally, intermittent fasting helps you not to lose that much muscle compared to just fasting. When you still have some type of muscle on your body, your muscles work harder than fat to increase your metabolism, so you are losing weight while doing limited activities. When your muscles are used to this time of method of eating, you are essentially eating your way to losing weight, which is extremely helpful in the long-term of trying to maintain a healthy weight and healthy lifestyle. Another hormone that is affected by intermittent fasting is leptin. This hormone tells your brain which then tells your body when you are hungry. If you are obese, this hormone is overactive. Your body reads this hunger cue no matter if you are hungry or not which cause you to overeat. Thus, extra food and energy make you gain weight. When you fast, it helps improve your leptin sensitivity, so your body is more in tune with your hunger triggers, like ghrelin. Intermittent fasting sends your brain more measured indicators of your hunger, so you are not overeating. However, it is important to stick to a pattern of fasting, especially if you are intermittent fasting, to avoid an increase of cortisol, which can lead to more stress or insomnia if you are not consistent with your fasting window.

Intermittent fasting also prevents insulin resistance. Some people with Type 2 diabetes who have consulted with their physician even intermittent fast to help control their diabetes. Diabetes is a chronic illness that occurs when a person's body is not able to send glucose, or blood sugar to your body. Glucose is what your body eat and in order to get that glucose your body needs insulin. People with type 1 diabetes do not produce insulin at all. Whereas people with type 2 diabetes produce insulin, but their bodies don't use insulin as efficiently as it should. As type 2 diabetes progresses, people tend not to make insulin at all. Dr. Jason Fung did a study where 3 men fasted for a time frame of 10 months. Two of the men fasted every other day. And one man fasted three days a week. On the days that the men fasted, they were able to have low-calorie drinks like coffee, tea, and water. They could also have one low-calorie meal. At the end of the study, two of the men did not take any of their diabetes drugs. The last man had stopped taking four out of the five drugs that he was taking to control his diabetes. Dr. Fung asserts that fasting can be helpful for those with type 2 diabetes. However, other doctors caution against people taking this study as the complete truth since the study was only limited to three people. Nevertheless, the results seem quite promising. The most important thing from this study was Dr. Jason Fung demonstrated that fasting does have a positive effect on controlling diabetes. In the future, fasting will most likely be used as an important way to regulate, if not cure, type 2 diabetes. An important consideration before fasting it to remember that if you are taking medication for your type 2 diabetes, you need to check in with your physician before attempting to fast to control your type 2 diabetes.

Additionally, intermittent fasting is great in reducing the risks of heart disease. Based on studies with animals, intermittent fasting improves the markers for certain diseases that give you heart disease. When the animals intermittently fasted, their blood pressure, triglycerides, inflammatory and cholesterol levels went down, which means that their risk for heart disease went down, too. When practicing intermittent fasting, the animals have improved in all these categories. This looks very promising for humans as well. Another major reason people are attracted to intermittent fasting is because of its preventative characteristics. Intermittent fasting also helps to stabilize your glucose levels as well since it helps regulate your insulin, glucagon, and blood glucose levels. This regulation helps your body regulate how your body uses the sugar you eat during the day. If this process goes more efficiently, your body has no choice but to burn weight more efficiently as well. Intermittent fasting, coupled with the reduced risk of getting diabetes, also helps your body get rid of inflammation. What's one of the major causes of inflammation? Sugar, which when you are intermittently fasting is advised that you avoid. Inflammation is a factor behind lots of chronic diseases like diabetes, heart disease, asthma, and stomach issues. Intermittent fasting tackles these inflammation-causing factors and helps a person improve and heal themselves from inflammatory diseases. Moreover, intermittent fasting encourages the limiting of sugar in your daily diet. A diet full of whole foods packed with macronutrients and electrolytes is suggested when you fast instead of sugary, junk food. This focus on eating healthily along with passing you the key tenets of intermittent fasting. When your body is able to fight inflammation effectively, it helps improve your immune system. So intermittent fasting creates a healthy domino effect in your body that fights fat, inflammation, improves your immune system, and prevents chronic disease at the same time.

Intermittent fasting is great for your brain because it helps prevent an increase in a hormone found in your brain called brain-derived neurotrophic factor or (BDNF). When you have an overabundance of this hormone, you could potentially be at risk for having depressing. Intermittent fasting helps your brain create new fresh brain cells to clean out the BDNF hormones. Your heart is another beneficiary of the intermittent lifestyle. Based on studies with animals, intermittent fasting improves the markers for certain diseases that give you heart disease. When the animals intermittently fasted, their blood pressure, triglycerides, inflammatory and cholesterol levels went down, which means that their risk for heart disease went down, too. When practicing intermittent fasting, the animals have improved in all these categories. This looks very promising for humans as well.

On the horizon, there also seems to be steady streams of information that points to intermittent fasting helping seizures, another brain disease. The reason intermittent fasting helps with epilepsy is that it helps repair the problematic cells in your brain that cause seizures. Intermittent fasting coupled with a ketogenic diet has done wonders for those with seizures. The ketogenic diet does not allow for candy or high-carbohydrate foods, like pasta, rice, and bread. The food in this diet is also weighed carefully on a diet scale before consuming. This diet is also beneficial for those that do not have seizures. Since 1995, thousands of papers have been produced to show that intermittent fasting is a viable option to help him reduce his seizures.

Intermittent fasting is also one of the best anti-aging agents around due to its ability to reduce your stress hormone levels and keep your liver healthy. Another reason people choose to fast is to improve their physical appearance. Fasting reduces oxidative stress. To fully understand how oxidative stress works, there first must be a quick definition of what free radicals are. Free radicals are atoms in your body that are unstable. In order to get stable, the free radicals have to join two other substances in your body to get stable. When free radicals join with other substances in your body, it causes oxidative stress. Hence, oxidative stress can cause cells to break down in your body and can result in issues such as inflammation and wrinkles and diseases or even chronic diseases. When you fast, it helps your body prevent forming these free radicals that can destroy your body in so many ways. Intermittent fasting also increases the human growth hormone which increases your body's collagen production. More collagen means that your body will have younger-looking skin. Moreover, fasting increases the process of autophagy, which is how your body repairs itself by making newer and healthier cells. When you have newer and healthier cells, your skin improves. Fasting also helps the fluid that accumulates under the skin lessen, which also improves your overall appearance since salt is eliminated from your body when you fast. Less salt in your body increases your appearance and slows down the aging process.

The last major benefit of fasting that will be explored in this chapter is when people fast to improve their heart health. High blood pressure, cholesterol, diabetes, and obesity are all indicators of heart health problems. Fasting helps reduce all of these risks. However, fasting can cause an imbalance of your electrolytes, so when a person fasts, they must make sure that they are consuming enough electrolytes not to affect their heart health negatively. More about electrolytes will be discussed later in the book.

Additionally, intermittent fasting helps improve your physical experience and helps your body get rid of waste more efficiently. Your cells are constantly using the nutrients in your body that you get from and getting rid of the waste. This process of getting rid of waste is called autography. As a person ages, Autophagy becomes more and more difficult to activate. However, not eating for at least 12 hours or more helps the body's tissues and cells to clean themselves. Increasing glucagon which is what happens when we deny our body of nutrients helps increase autophagy. For women, sometimes their body's response to autophagy is not as strong as men. So intermittent fasting may not be as strong a trigger for jumpstarting autophagy if that's your goal for some women. As a matter of fact, some disease takes advantage or the process of autophagy and use it to kill healthy cells. These types of diseases tend to affect men more since fasting can cause the autophagy process to slow down in some women. For men or women, if their body has a difficult time getting rid of waste well, it can lead to diseases like Alzheimer's and cancer. Guess what helps your body rid itself of the waste more efficiently? That's right – intermittent fasting. Intermittent fasting has also helped improve your cognitive functions and helping you stay sharp by increasing epinephrine & norepinephrine levels.

Research seems to suggest that intermittent fasting can help you live longer. The constant healing effects that intermittent fasting has on your body helps your body reset daily in a more efficient and helpful way to improve your overall quality and life. This conclusion is also supported by studies done on animals. The animals that intermittently fasted every other day lived about 80% longer than animals that did not. Intermittent fasting is ideal for a plethora of health reasons. Some extremists even claim that intermittent fasting is the key to everlasting Youth and perhaps even immortality. While all these claims have not been verified, there are lots of benefits that intermittent fasting brings that can help you maintain a healthier life for longer. Hopefully, this chapter has given you more insight into how intermittent fasting can be beneficial to your life. Since we have the science behind us, it's time to move on to the fun part. Now it's time to explore the different intermittent fasting protocols you can choose to adopt in your life.

Chapter 5: Various Intermittent Fasting Protocols

Hands down, the best part about intermittent fasting is the ability to choose which protocol you want to follow. You can try different protocols until you find the one that works for you. Intermittent fasting does not require you to eat exotic ingredients or adhere to strict dietary rules. It is this flexibility of intermittent fasting that allows you to continue to have a social life and enjoy your food. It's not a hard-and-fast extreme diet so even if you slip up you have the ability to pick right back up the next day. It is this gentle approach and flexibility that makes intermittent fasting a favorite of many people.

Before you begin, make a deal to be kind to yourself. You will make mistakes, but it's up to you to correct them the best way you know how. Do not be alarmed if you ever run into bumps. This chapter will give you an idea of the different intermittent fasting protocols to choose from. We'll begin talking about intermittent fasting first. Intermittent fasting is eating during certain windows and then not eating during other windows. It may sound complicated, but it's really not. Most people have done some sort of fasting without even knowing.

The easiest way to practice intermittent fasting is to skip the meal that is easiest for you according to your current schedule. This version is called spontaneous fasting. Maybe you are in a rush and forget to eat breakfast. You just intermittently fasted! Perhaps you are preparing for a busy meeting and decide to skip lunch. Yup, you just intermittently fasted. Spontaneous intermittent fasting is very easy to do, and many often partake in it without knowing it. To make this method more effective, instead of missing a meal by accident, you will miss it purposefully. If you are already doing this accidentally, then you can just fine tune it so it can become your official intermittent fasting method. This is definitely one of the easiest methods to do since it happens without you thinking about it. However, there are other methods that you can definitely consider, as well.

One of the most popular methods of intermittent fasting is called the lean-gains method. This is where you fast for fourteen hours and eat in a 10 hour window period. This method of intermittent fasting is coupled with intense training as a way to lose weight quicker. Another popular variation is called the 16/8 fast. While you do this type of fast, you only eat during an 8 to 10-hour window and then you fast the other 16 hours of the day. Popular times to fast can be from 10 am to 6 pm, or 9 am to 5 pm, or even 11 am to 7 pm. This method of fasting is beneficial because you are able to follow your natural hunger cycles. Some people are never hungry in the morning, so they are able to forgo breakfast. Some people do not like to eat after a certain amount of time in the evening, so they forego dinner. By using this method of fasting, you are able to add intermittent fasting to your lifestyle without having to make a major adjustment. To take this method to the next level, some people fast for 20 hours and only eat during a 4-hour window.

The next version of intermittent fasting is called The Warrior Diet. When you practice this version of intermittent fasting, you only eat small pieces of raw fruits and vegetables during the day and eat one major meal at night. The major meal you eat should be limited to about 500-600 calories for women and 800-900 calories for men. Muslims practice a form of this intermittent fasting version during Ramadan when they forgo eating during the day and only eat after sunset.

Every other day fasting is when you fast every other day. During this version of fasting, you eat a limited amount of meals during your off days and on the days that you are allowed to eat you just eat regularly. A similar version of this intermittent fasting method is called the 5:2. During this method, you eat for 5 full days, and you fast for 2 days by only eating a total of 500 to 600 calories on the days that you are fasting. For women, if you are using this method, it is advised that you eat 500 calories, and for men, it is advised that you eat 600 calories. You can break your smaller meals into two meals of 300 calories or 250 calories respectively. The trick when using this method is to eat the same amount as you would if you were eating regularly on the days that you can eat. You also do not want to fast for two days in a row, especially for women. It is advised that you break up the fasting days during the week so that the two fasting days are not one after the other.

With this intermittent fasting method, it is extremely important to meal plan to make sure that you are reaching your caloric limit. This method requires that you are vigilant about your meal planning so that you are not overeating or undereating. This method can definitely be more challenging to start with, but once you get into the habit of doing it, it will become a lot easier.

The more you fast, the more you can potentially lose weight as long as you are making sure that you are eating healthy during your eating times. One of the most difficult intermittent fasting methods is called the 24-hour fast or the Up Day, Down Day Fasting method. Some people fast from dinner one day to the end of the next day or breakfast one day to breakfast the next day. For beginners, it is probably best to start off with a smaller window and work your way up to not eating for longer periods of time. Only the most advanced, most determined fasters should try this initially. This method also requires lots of willpower and self-control. Those new to intermittent fasting might read this and think, "Who in the world is trying this method of intermittent fasting?" Sure, actors and actresses may use this method to get ready for movie roles, but a lot of regular people use it, too. You will be surprised that it is very convenient for lots of people to follow. As you become more versed with intermittent fasting, you may find that you too that prefer The Warrior Diet over different methods of intermittent fasting.h

Overall, a 24-hour fast is great for giving your physical body a reset. It helps reset your system for issues related to your appetite, gut, and energy. When you begin this fast, you want to still go through your regular routine. When your fasting for 24 hours or longer, try to stay away from food so you won't be tempted and try to keep your mind clear from thinking about food. Remember, anyone can fast up to three days without any medical supervision. If you are doing an alternate day fast or a 5:2 fast, you can slowly transition to going to one full day of not eating.

The night before you begin your fast is very important, so make sure that you are eating a balanced meal. Get up and start your day like normal. You can even start off with tea or water or coffee. And go through your regular activities. By the time you finish, you will notice that your 24 hours have gone by quickly. Once it's time to break the fast, don't just eat a huge meal. Slowly ease into the meal, so you don't get sick. Start off by drinking a nice warm glass of lemon water that will prepare your stomach for the coming meal. Wait thirty minutes and then have a low carb snack. Wait another thirty minutes and then eat a nice, well-balanced meal. Also, don't overdo the meal. After any fast, do not eat everything you see to avoid gaining unnecessary weight. Control your urges so you can get the most out of your fast. Also, don't be alarmed if you have to go to the bathroom more after you fast. It's your body's natural reaction to your higher metabolism that may occur after a fast. You can take a probiotic before eating to try and regulate your urge.

A 36-Hour Fast

A 36-hour fast is extremely helpful for those who have type 2 diabetes due to their higher insulin resistance compared to those with type 1 diabetes. For this type of fast, it is recommended that a person does it 2-3 times a week for those with type 2 diabetes. People who don't have diabetes will also benefit from this fast. One of the easiest ways to do it is to have dinner around 6 or 7 pm on Day 1. On Day 2, you wouldn't eat any meals, only drink fluids with no calories added. Then you wouldn't eat until 6 or 7 am on the third day. It may feel weird at first, but this type of fast is definitely doable.

A 42-Hour Fast

A 42-hour fast builds on the 36-hour fast. You would still have dinner around 6 pm on Day 1. On Day 2, you wouldn't eat any meals, only drink fluids with no calories added. Then you wouldn't eat until noon on the third day. An easy way to transition into a 42-hour fast is to get into the habit of having your first meal around noon-time. To start this habit, in the morning, you would wake up and have a cup of coffee or water. If you get into the habit of having your first meal around noon, your body won't feel as hungry when you first wake up.

It is important to remember that when you are doing a longer fast, you don't want to restrict your calories. Eat normal sized meals, but don't overdo it. You may think that you will want to eat everything in sight once you finish your fast, but you may realize that your appetite goes down. So eating until you are full does not result in a huge feast like expected.

A Two-Week Fast

A two-weeks fasting protocol builds on all the other fasts. It's essentially water fast for 2 weeks. Before beginning this type of fast, you want to prepare. Before you begin, take the time to detox from unhealthy foods and habits like smoking and not getting enough sleep. The food selections you will want to avoid are dairy, sugar, alcohol, eggs, fish, caffeinated drinks and meat. Try to eat raw foods every day for about a week before to make the longer fat easier to maintain.

After you have prepared, you can start the time to fast. You may be hungry but resist the urge to eat. The desire for hunger normally passes after three days. Stay hydrated to help you get through this stage. It's at this stage that people begin to think clearer and feel empowered. While staying hydrated, you also want to make sure you are taking your electrolytes. You can take them via supplements. You'll want to have magnesium, phosphate, calcium, potassium, and sodium. You will want to check with your preferred medical provider before embarking upon such a fast. A two-week can go fast quickly, and you can trigger fatal symports if you are not prepared properly. You may also experience extreme mood swings, so give your friends and family the heads up.

As you get deeper into the fast, you will start to feel fatigued, even dizziness, and sometimes blurred vision. Your breath can smell bad, and you may even get sick. This is your body's detox process. It shows that your body is responding well to the fast by getting rid of the toxins in your body. You may even experience some flu-like symptoms, like pains, aches, chills, and fevers. This is just your body's way of getting rid of the toxins by pushing them through your intestines, skins, lungs, nose, and stomach.

As some point, you will overcome the plateau. You will feel normal. You may even go back in forth between feeling sick and feeling normal. Again, this is your body responding positively to the fast. Stick it out if you can. If you notice any of the extreme symptoms from earlier in the book, that's when you want to reach out to your medical provider. If you can make it through a 2-week fast, you will feel amazed afterward.

For this type of fast, do not try to work out - just take it easy. Be thoughtful and meditate. To make it through the fast, you can stay in airy and bright rooms. When you fast, your body may give off an odor so this will help dissipate quicker. The bright room will improve your mood. Also, try to take in the sun for about 10 to 20 minutes daily before it gets too hot. To help with your breath, brush your tongue with activated charcoal powder. You can also scrub your skin with a dry brush and bathe multiple times a day to keep the odor at bay. To take the fast to another level, you can take two enemas daily during the first week and only once until the fast is over. One of the most important things is to surround yourself with people who care if you're going to make it. They will help you get through the tough times.

When it's time to break the fast, go extremely slow. The longer you go without food, the longer you need to spend slowly reintroducing the food back into your life. You can start with bone broth and then small meals. Don't try to eat everything at once. Go slowly. Most people prefer intermittent fasting, but a longer fast has immense health and spiritual or mental benefits. Ultimately, it's up to you to decide if an extended fast is best for you or not.

Another popular intermittent fasting, one that has the most research done on it, is every other day fast, or alternate daily fasting (ADF). Don't let the name fool you. Alternate daily fasting is similar to the 5:2 diet in that you can eat up to 500 calories on the days that you fast. The only difference is that you fast on alternate days rather than twice a week like in the 5:2 diets. Intermittent fasting is usually less than 24 hours, but there are those who have had smashing success with longer diets, specifically, 24-hour, 36-hour, 42-hour, and 2 weeks fasts. You will be surprised that the longer one fasts, the less hungry they get. You will also realize that longer fasts are not impossible, and if you can successfully get through one, you may realize how awesome it is. We will talk about longer fasts in the next chapter.

For women, the best way to fast without throwing their hormones out of whack is to try to fast for 12 to 16 hours a day on two to three non-consecutive days. On the days that they fast, try to do light cardio or yoga. More intense workouts like strength or HIIT training can be done on the non-fasting days. Be sure to drink lots of liquids like tea, water, and coffee. If you are drinking tea and coffee, try not to put any sweetener or milk in it. You can also try to add a few amino acid supplements. If you feel comfortable, after 2 weeks, you can try to add another day of fasting. Not every woman is the same, and the results may vary per women.

For women, it is important to go slowly and gradually to prevent adverse effects. Remember, you are not Superwoman or Superman, so take it slow to prevent hurting yourself and the people who care about you. Some people even like the form support groups of other minted fasters to encourage each other to keep going. This is especially helpful on the days that you want to work out. Exercising with others who understand what you're going through and who are going through the same thing with you can be empowering, encouraging, and helpful as you tried to stay the intermittent fasting path. Other still like to hire a trainer that is familiar with intermittent fasting to make sure if they are tapping into the best workout that can leverage the intermittent fasting lifestyle. Whether you want to work out by yourself or with others on YouTube or in person or with a trainer, it is advisable that you continue to work out and do not give up exercise just because you are intermittent fasting. Exercising is still part of having a healthy lifestyle.

When you are intermittent fasting, it is important to pay attention to your body! Keep a food journal if you can. (You can buy one online or use a digital one.) A person should always be aware of the effects intermittent fasting is having on their body. You will know that your body is not responding positively to intermittent fasting. If at any time, you notice these things, you should stop.

- **Insomnia** – If you are consistently staying up all night, and just can't sleep, then you need to stop intermittent fasting, so you look into the root cause of your insomnia further.
- **Extreme hunger to the point that you can't do anything else unless you are thinking about food.** – Intermittent fasting should be easy to do. Yes, at times, you will feel hunger. However, you should not be thinking about food so much that you are not able to function. There are a few tips you can use to alleviate your hunger pangs in Chapter 6 that can help you make it through your fasting windows. The truth of the matter once you get used to your fasting window, making it won't be an issue. The only concern you should have is if you can't make it through the intermittent fasting window and you cannot function AT ALL.
- **Weight gain, specifically in your mid-area.** – Unexpected weight gain, which usually is the opposite effect of intermittent fasting should be cause for concern. If at any point, you notice unexpected weight gain, you should definitely reach out to your doctor.
- **Your period goes away or changes.** – For women, this is extremely important. If you notice any abnormal changes to your period while fasting, you may need to stop. Long term issues with your period could cause fertility issues so if you notice anything, speak out. If you think your ovulation is at risk or you feel like you are running into fertility issues, please, please, please reach out to your doctor.
- **You are especially stressed out.** – Intermittent fasting surprisingly helps people gain mental clarity. However, if you feel utterly and completely overwhelmed, it is ok to stop fasting, especially if you

have low energy and can't concentrate. If you feel that your performance has declined tremendously because of fasting, do not be afraid to stop.

- **Skin and hair health** – If you notice that your skin's color looks off your hair seems thinner and brittle, this is a cause for concern. Any drastic changes with your hair and skin is an important indication that intermittent fasting isn't working.

- **Decreased bone density and muscle tone decreases**. – A change in your muscles or pain in your muscles can be a cause for concern. If you notice that your muscle tone has decreased or you feel pains doing your regular actions like walking the steps or getting in and out of cars, then you may want to reach out to your primary physician.

- **You begin to have a change in digestion.** – If at any point, you notice that you are having digestion issues that you were not having before, then intermittent fasting could be the cause. If there is extreme discomfort to where you cannot function, then reach out to your doctor. Some change in your digestion schedule is expected. However, if you notice something is way off, call the doctor.

- **You are always cold.** – Extreme coldness is another indication that you need to stop intermittent fasting. If you are colder than usual, and you have done everything you can to stay warm, but just can't stay warm. Then you need to reach out to your doctor.

The good news is that it is not all doom and gloom. However, there is a way to effectively practice intermittent fasting without falling into this vicious cycle, which is to begin fasting gradually. Do not begin all at once to prevent your body from going out of whack. More attention will be given to this in the next chapter. Ultimately, if you pay attention to your body, you will be able to tell if intermittent fasting is for you or not. Trust your body and listen carefully. If you let you know, so you do not have to be scared to try. Using the tips in this book will help you ease into the journey, so your body is not shell-shocked.

When you fast, you need to also pay attention to the electrolytes that you are consuming. Electrolytes are the chemicals our bodies need to survive a fasted state. Electrolytes are already coming in our daily diet, but special attention should be given to them when you fast to make sure you are meeting your nutrient requirements in spite of fasting. Meeting the requirements are usually easy to do. As a matter of fact, most of us meet them every day without a hitch, but it is great to know what they are so you can be better prepared to handle intermittent fasting. After water, the most important ones are:

- **Calcium** – This is found in leafy greens like collard greens, spinach, kale and sardines, and dairy. You will know you have calcium deficiency if you have muscle spasms or bone issues.
- **Potassium** – This electrolyte can be found in bananas, plain yogurt, and potato skins. If you have mental confusion, weakness of the muscles or paralysis of the muscles, you may have a deficiency.
- **Magnesium** – Found in pumpkin seeds, spinach, and halibut, it is important to have this electrolyte. Confusion, nausea or muscle cramps are an indicator that you may be deficient in this electrolyte.
- **Sodium** – This electrolyte is in soup, salt, tomato juice, dill pickles, and tomato sauce. You know you

may need this electrolyte if you have a loss of appetite or muscle cramps or dizziness.

- **Chloride** – If you have an irregular heartbeat or changes in your pH, you may be experiencing a deficiency in these electrolytes. It is found in veggies like tomatoes, olives, lettuce and table salt.

The most important electrolytes to have while fasting is magnesium, potassium, and sodium. You should have about a teaspoon of salt a day and mix it with water; 2000 milligrams of potassium and at least 300 to 450 milligrams of magnesium. When you are eating, as long as you are eating foods rich in these electrolytes it can sustain you during the fasted stated. Eating healthy during your eating windows is just as important as not eating during your fasting periods. If at some point you feel comfortable with intermittent fasts, you can consider moving to extended fasts, starting with at least 24-hours.

Choose Your Intermittent Fasting Method

Before you decide which method you want to use, the first thing you need to do before you begin intermittent fasting is to determine why you want to begin in the first place. Are you doing intermittent fasting in order to lose weight? Are you doing intermittent fasting to lead a healthier lifestyle? Are you doing intermittent fasting for another specific health outcome, like to lower your blood pressure or cholesterol levels or to even increase your metabolism or energy? Whatever your reason is before beginning, make that reason clear so you can always come back to it as a point of reference when you feel like you are getting weak at any moment.

While your weight loss and health journey are different than other people's, it is interesting to look at other people who intermittent fast to see what they're doing and what works for them. You can use them as inspiration. You can also form your own support group to hold you accountable for your reasons for intermittent fasting. You can find this support group online or in person, like a family member or trusted friend. Checking out online boards every now and then is also great to do in order to keep your info up-to-date and to recharger your intermittent fasting battery.

The next thing you want to do before you begin is to speak with your doctor. When you meet, let your doctor know what your reasons for wanting to do intermittent fasting are. Then see if they have any input. This especially important if you have diabetes, are elderly or pregnant or have a history of eating disorders.

The next important step you should do before you begin is to have realistic expectations. If you plan on losing 50 pounds in a week, that's most likely not going to happen. It is healthy to lose at least two pounds a week. Even if you have a realistic expectation of how much weight you want to lose, what happens if you are not seeing the results you think you should be seeing? (We'll talk about this some in the next chapter.)

The most important point about your expectations is to adjust them. You may not meet your expectations, and that is ok. You can adjust your expectations or adjust your actions to meet them. Do not get discouraged if you do not meet your expectations. Keep going! You do not want to throw in the towel too soon or throw the towel in without adjusting your expectations. No matter what your expectations are, continue to arm yourself with the proper information by researching so, you can see how intermittent fasting best fits into your lifestyle. When you have your reasons for doing intermittent fasting and your food journal ready, you can go ahead and begin.

Schedule your Day of Reckoning. This is the day where you get rid of everything in your kitchen that's not going to help you with your intermittent fasting journey. These items are things like junk food, alcohol, snacks, salty and sugary drinks. Sugary drinks include diet drinks and health drinks like Gatorade or Powerade. These all contain fructose which is just as deadly and inflammation causing as sugar. You can give those bad foods to a friend or family member, a food bank or just throw them away. For the more dramatic people like me, you can even burn them.

Next thing is, like Nike, 'Just do it!' Pick your fasting window and eating time and start. Initially, do not expect just to go 24 hours without food, definitely build up to that goal. When you start off slow, you can try to avoid maybe eating breakfast since you already sleeping and coming from a fast. Another way to get a slow start is if you try to reduce the portions of a certain food that you're eating before you totally give up the food that you're eating. For example, if you just have to have 10 cokes a day. Trying have 5, then 3, then 1, until you are at zero.

Other ways to go incrementally fast are to change perhaps the portion of the food that you're eating. If you are used to eating carbohydrate-heavy meals, slowly change your diet to include more fruits and vegetables until your portions start to consist of mostly vegetables and whole foods. If you eat more white bread or grain products, work on not eating them or even substituting them for healthier options like sprouted bread or wheat or brown carbohydrates. This incremental beginning can help you be more successful when you ramp up to more intense versions of intermittent fasting such as skipping days at a time.

Remember, before you begin an extended fast, make sure you have consulted with a medical professional and are comfortable with your reasons for partaking upon the fast. Once you have this figured out, you will be able to move to prepare for the fast. You should know that extended fasting is perfectly safe and will cause you to reevaluate how you think of hunger. By the time you finish with your extended fast, you will no longer think of hunger as a negative.

Daresay, you may think of it as a way to improve your mental health. And accept hunger for what it is – a brief moment that you can master. When you decide to do an extended fast, do not be afraid hunger, rather figure out ways to master it. However, start off slow and build longer. Just keep in mind that this is a marathon and not a sprint. You're building healthy habits for a lifetime so don't feel pressured to rush right out the gate. For the people who may think that you are crazy, don't put any stock into their thoughts. If you know your "why" of doing intermittent fasting, then you have nothing to worry about. Stay focused on your long-term goal and let everything else fall by the wayside.

Chapter 6: Cautions While Making the Transition to Intermittent Fasting

It cannot be overemphasized the importance of paying attention to your body while fasting can be. You don't have to be perfect as an intermittent faster, but you do want to pay attention to your body and the signs it is giving you. Fasting is indeed a lifestyle, and there are a few mistakes you want to be aware of once you begin. Knowing what they are beforehand will hopefully help you not to have to struggle with them at all. Even if you run into any bumps in the road, remember to get right back up and to keep going. You are not expected to be perfect the first time you try your hand at. With careful planning and perseverance, you will be intermittent fasting like a pro in no time.

These are some of the top mistakes that people make while they are intermittent fasting. Take notes and try to avoid them if you can.

- **Over-eating and binge-eating** – Avoiding overeating and binge-eating during your time to eat is important. When it is time to eat, eat a regular sized portion and do not try to compensate for your fasting period. This overcompensation prevents you from taking advantage of your intermittent fasting period.
- **Not eating enough** - When you eat, do not feel like you can't eat. Take advantage of your eating period, but do not gorge yourself. Make sure you are eating healthy food and not junk. If you make sure your food is full of macronutrients, you will be able to make it

through your fasted states easier.

- **Not drinking enough water** – Water is the life force of us all and staying hydrated is a major key to making the intermittent lifestyle work for you. Staying hydrated prevents cravings and helps you make it through the fasting period. Do not neglect this important step.

- **Not choosing the right method** – Intermittent fasting should be easy. If it feels like you have to work too much or it is not flowing with your lifestyle, do not be afraid to try a new method. There is not a hard and fast rule about which method is the best. Whichever method you choose should fit into your lifestyle. Remember, this is a lifestyle change and not a diet. You can take the time to figure out which method works the best for you.

- **Obsessing too much** - If you are weighing yourself obsessively or worrying about if you are doing intermittent fasting, take a deep breath and relax. Results can take time. You shouldn't expect a drastic change overnight; just relax and take your time. Before you know it, you will see the benefits that are extremely helpful.

- **Giving up too soon** – Do not join the many other people who threw in the towel too soon on intermittent fasting. Give yourself about two weeks to measure the results and see if it is working or not. Do not just give up after a day or two. This method is proven throughout time to work. This tricky part is finding which method works out the best for you. Keep playing around with it and do not give up too soon. However, if, at any point, you experience drastic results, it may be time to throw in the towel.

Ultimately, if you are food journaling, you will be able to pick up on some of these mistakes that you make. Any time you noticed a mistake, try to find a way to correct it with better practice. Be gentle and kind to yourself and keep going. You will soon realize that intermittent fasting and fasting is not that bad.

While the intermittent fasting benefits are numerous for both men and women, it is important to note that intermittent fasting benefits women in different ways than men.

Due to our biological makeup, fasting affects women's bodies differently than it affects men's bodies. Certain reactions to fasting are more pronounced in women's bodies than and men's body. This is not to say that women or men should not do intermittent fasting, they should. However, they need to be aware of the potential differences that can occur when you begin intermittent fasting that is dependent upon if you are a man or woman. This is not written to scare you but just to cause you to be aware of said differences. Before a woman begins to intermittent fast, she needs to do a self-examination.

To truly get the maximum benefits and to organically maximize the benefits, she needs to ask herself a few questions. (Men can ask themselves these questions too as it will apply to them somewhat, but these are important concerns that women definitely need to ask themselves.)

- **Are you getting enough sleep?** – This question is important because if you are not getting enough sleep, the intermittent fasting can have negative effects on your body. Intermittent fasting is supposed to help you improve your sleep.

- **Are you already on a calorie-restricted diet and lean?** – This is an important question to ask because if a woman is already pretty lean and is restricting her calories, intermittent fasting can trigger a more adverse effect and be too strong for her body. This extra restriction can send her body past the gluconeogenesis state and trigger the starvation mode.
- **How much are you exercising?** – If you are already exercising an intense amount of time, intermittent fasting again may have adverse effects because you are pushing your body to starvation mode. Since everyone's body is different, there is not a hard and fast rule, as long as you are exercising not too little and not too much, you should be ok.
- **Why do you want to intermittent fast?** – If you want to try it because you are obese and need to lose with, or your neurologist says its ok to help prevent dementia or other types of cognitive decline, or you need to improve the benefits of chemotherapy, sure thing. However, if you are trying to do it to increase weight loss from an intense exercise schedule or you want to go from already ok body weight to a smaller one or prevent pregnancy weight, you may want to pause. Intermittent fasting should be healthy and make sense, not an extreme lifestyle choice that you cannot bear.

Intermittent fasting can throw a woman's hormones balance off if she does not pay attention to her body. Since women can produce babies, our bodies are already very sensitive to our hunger cues. If a woman's body feels that she is being starved, she will begin to make more ghrelin or leptin which hunger hormones are. If a woman ignores these cues, her body makes more of those hormones, and if you ignore them, it can cause ovulation to stop or even shrink ovaries, which prevents periods and can cause overeating and eating disorders.

Intermittent fasting also has the potential to throw your estrogen out of balance as well. While hormone imbalance is a concern for many people, especially women, when they begin to intermittent fast, the good thing to keep in mind is that you will definitely know if something is wrong because your body will let you know. Remember, that intermittent fasting should fit your temperament, lifestyle, and personality. Do not feel like you have to be committed to only one type of intermittent fasting protocol. You are in the driver's seat of your healthy lifestyle so you can change the direction you're going at any time. You aren't a failure if you do so; rather, you are being a boss and taking charge of the life you want to live.

Chapter 7: Common Myths About Intermittent Fasting

At this point, I am sure that you have a lot of questions that you need to be answered about fasting and myths that need to be busted. For those who are on the fence or those who are excited to begin, this section will be especially helpful. It will go over some common myths that may give you pause before beginning as well as alleviate some of the fears you may have. Hopefully, by the time you finish reading, you will be ready to get started fasting!

Is it safe?

Yes. For healthy adults, intermittent fasting should not be an issue. You may even realize that there are many more benefits to intermittent fasting than you thought. However, for those who are elderly, pregnant, breastfeeding or taking medication, check with your healthcare provider first.

Will I start to starve?

Gandhi was able to go on a hunger strike, only drinking water, and did not die. A few extended hours between meals is not going to cause you to starve or die. Our bodies normally have about a month's worth of stored fat available to us every day. So you will have a constant energy supply even if you intermittently fast.

How do I get over the mental block of not eating?

If you do not eat, you feel like you are starving. Ever had this feeling? No worries, you are not alone. This is a common feeling to have. Sometimes when we get that feeling, it doesn't mean that we're always hungry. It can mean that you are thirsty instead. If you are having trouble overcoming this barrier, think about what you can do when you do get this feeling. What's your plan of action going to be? How about drinking a glass of water, listening to your favorite song or doing your favorite activity until the feeling passes? I'll be honest. The mental block of not being able to eat is one of the most difficult barriers overcome when doing intermittent fasting, but it is not difficult to overcome once you get in the habit of doing it. Once you make it through, you will realize that it will get easier and easier until your body gets used to the fasting period and your eating period.

There are a lot of questions that people have about intermittent fasting and the validity of how it can help improve your overall health. This chapter addresses some of the most common misconceptions and frequently asked questions one may have about intermittent fasting. Hopefully, after reading this chapter, if you are on the fence, you will be convinced about the positives about intermittent fasting.

What's the best diet to couple intermittent fasting with?

Great question. There is not an 'official' one. It depends on your goals. If you want to lose more weight, popular diets to pair with intermittent fasting are vegan, vegetarian or keto diets. More important than diet is the importance of eating a well-balanced diet not matter which dietary option you decide upon and stay within our caloric limits.

Can I use the ketogenic diet to intermittent fast if I am diabetic?

Some people have coupled intermittent fasting with a keto diet with some success. However, there are still studies being done to determine if this is the best way to do intermittent fasting with diabetes. There are some benefits to intermittent fasting with diabetes like regulation of your insulin and glycogen levels. However, the most important step is to talk with your healthcare provider before deciding to take this journey.

How much can I train on an empty stomach?

The most difficult part of training while intermittent fasting is to let your body get used to it. When your body gets used to working out while fasting, you will realize that you may get extra strength and energy to do your workout. When you train while you fast, your workout can be more efficient and help you burn more calories or build more muscle. So if you can handle training on an empty stomach go for it. Ultimately, it is up to you and your exercise goals to decide what you can handle.

Many people decide to train during their eating window so they can eat a pre and post workout meal. If you are trying to lose weight, foregoing your pre-workout meal will tremendously help. Just remember that after your work out, try to eat protein and fiber to rebuild your body from the workout. Others also find that eating more carbohydrates on the days that they work out, helps them with the workouts.

Can I just eat fruits as a main meal?

It is best to eat a balanced diet. Too much fruit could give you too much sugar and give you unwanted weight gain if you do it too often. If you prefer fruits, try to disguise your greens by adding your greens with your fruits in a juice blend or smoothie.

What are the side effects?

You may experience headaches, diarrhea, cramps, and discomfort. You may also experience insomnia, lower back pain, and hair loss. But if you experience these, reach out to your health care providers since these are extreme side effects. The most common side effects are hunger pangs, headaches, and discomfort. You should not feel totally lethargic or as if you cannot function by missing a meal or two a day. If you try intermittent fasting and you have just horrible side effects, it may not be for you, and that is okay.

How do I help with my hunger pangs?

One way to help with your hunger is to drink lots of liquid especially water. You can drink a big glass of water when you wake up or anytime you experience hunger pangs. What's more, you can put Himalayan salt in your water to give it an extra boost. You can also drink tea, amino acids, and coffee as much as you'd like, too. Just watch the extras like milk, cream, and sugar.

How can I tell if intermittent fasting or fasting is working?

One way to tell if it is working or not is to look at your body. Are you losing weight? How do you feel? Do you feel like you are sleeping better? Do you have a clearer mind or energy boost? Do you feel happiness generally? These are factors to look at when deciding if it is the right lifestyle for you or not. It is also important to note which method of intermittent fasting works best for you.

Why should I skip breakfast? Is not breakfast the most important meal of the day?

Wonderful question. The word breakfast means to break the fast. This idea that breakfast is the most important meal of the day is from an outdated diet concept. The typical American diet consists of sugary breakfast options like waffles, pancakes, pastries, etc. If you are not going to eat a healthy breakfast, why eat it anyway? Making sure you have enough calories throughout the day is more important than when you eat it. So if you eat your first meal at lunch, then your 'breakfast' would be your 'lunch.'

Eating breakfast or not is totally up to your body and whether you and your body can handle it or not. The great thing is if you need breakfast to function, just make it a part of your eating window and make sure you are eating a healthy option for breakfast. Most people tend to skip breakfast, so that's why skipping breakfast is not a major issue for most people. However, listen to your body and do what's best for your body's natural cycle.

Is not it healthier to eat more meals throughout the day?

This is a great question, too. The nutrients in your food and the number of calories you are eating is more important than when you eat it. If your body responds to smaller meals through the day, go ahead. If your body responds more to larger meals, feel free to do so. It is more important to make sure that you are not overeating your daily caloric limit than when you eat those meals.

If you partake in intermittent fasting, will you develop an eating disorder?

Intermittent fasting is not about developing an extreme eating pattern. It is a controlled pattern of eating during a certain time and not eating during another time. It is best matched up to your natural eating habits. The foods you eat are nutrient dense, so they are oftentimes healthier eating options that the foods you already partake in eating. Most people who do intermittent fasting do not develop an eating disorder. They actually become healthier from this lifestyle. However, if you have a history of having an eating disorder or are concerned that you may develop one by beginning, consult your healthcare professional before beginning.

Does intermittent fasting or fasting cause you to overeat?

Interesting, when you begin intermittent fasting, the exact opposite tends to happen. Unless you are purposefully overeating, you will find that your appetite tends to change and you start to crave smaller portions. Remember, American portions are many times larger than what normal portions are across the world so the smaller portions would be considered normal portions worldwide.

Will I gain weight if I eat later in the day or late at night?

The best thing about intermittent fasting is that it fits into your lifestyle. You can choose to decide when to eat your meals. Of course, if you are eating lots of carbohydrates only, overeating and not eating vegetables or fruit with a late eating window, you may gain weight. The key is moderation and balance. If you are eating a normal portion at night, you should not see weight gain. Again, it depends on your body. Keep notes in your food journal to see how your body reacts to eating at a later window. If you are operating at a calorie deficit, you should be fine. The most important thing is not to overeat to avoid giving yourself a stomach ache and extra calories.

Will I lose a lot of muscle when I intermittent fast or fast?

When you eat, your body releases the nutrients you need steadily over time. Until you need to replenish nutrients from your next meal. Many people assume that fasting immediately causes muscle loss which is not the case at all. When you fast, remember you are still using the nutrients from your previous meal even if it was 16 to 20 hours ago. So realistically you will not lose an extreme amount of muscle mass just by fasting in a certain window. However, if you are having concerns or will have concerns about losing muscle for whatever reason, consult with your healthcare professional for a second option. The objective of intermittent fasting is to be healthy, empowered, and informed.

Hopefully, this chapter has been able to put a lot of your doubts and fears to rest. Feel confident in knowing that many people practice intermittent fasting all over the world safely and without any hitches. Our ancient ancestors did too as well, so you're in great company if you decide to start intermittent fasting.

As you continue to learn about intermittent fasting, you will be surprised that it is actually quite healthy and has lots of benefits. Most of the misconceptions about intermittent fasting are perpetuated by people who have not intermittent fasted a day in their life, so be careful about how you take advice about intermittent fasting from. A lot of your doubts and fears will be resolved once you start practicing intermittent fasting. You will be blown away by all the positive effects it has on your body, and your body and health will thank you for it.

Chapter 8: Four Pillars to Make Intermittent Fasting a Success or You

Intermittent fasting can be a success for you if you focus on four important pillars. If you have these foundational concepts down, intermittent fasting should be a breeze. These pillars are food, exercise, routine, and sleep.

Food

One of the major tricks of being successful at intermittent fasting is to make sure that you have meals prepared so you will not be tempted to eat things that aren't good for you or overeat. In order to get those meals prepared ahead of time, you will want to have a pantry of your necessities in order to get those meals planned, but you have no idea how to begin. The first thing we will discuss is the approach to take. The first approach is easy. Since you already eat certain foods on a daily basis, find healthier recipes for the meals that you are already eating.

The next way is to build your meals ahead of time. When planning a meal, you can try to have three different colors – a fruit, veggie, bean or a whole-wheat grain. You will also want to try to cook foods a healthy way like steaming, baking or roasting instead of frying and grilling. Cooking at home will definitely help you save more calories than eating out. (However, if you must eat out, look for the healthiest alternatives you can find.)

One way to prepare your meals ahead of time is to assemble the ingredients and freeze them. So when it is time to make your meal, you can thaw the ingredients and make them. Another way to prepare your meals ahead of time is to prepare your entire meal, like casseroles or easily freezable recipes, and then un-thaw them ahead of time and prepare them. As you start to fast more and more, you will discover what meals are your favorites and which meals are the easiest to prepare. To give you an idea of what types of healthy ingredients you can stock up on before you begin meal planning follows.

- **Proteins** - Beans, quinoa, lean meats, nuts, peanut butter or your favorite type of nut butter
- **Vegetables** – Kale, spinach, lettuce, broccoli, mixed veggies, (The more vegetables you have, the merrier!)
- **Fiber** – Oatmeal
- **Fruit** – Fresh, canned and frozen. Be careful of the sugar content in canned and frozen fruits to make sure unnecessary sugar is not being added.
- **Healthy fats** – Nuts, seeds, olive oil and coconut oil, oily fish like salmon and tuna
- **Carbohydrates** – brown rice, wheat, and sprouted bread
- **Vitamins** – Fish oil, Vitamin C, your favorite brand of all-purpose vitamins

Other quick notes to remember are:

- Snacks and drinks add extra calories to your meal so be mindful of what you are eating and drinking throughout the day. Are you eating and drinking because you are hungry or because you are bored?

- Make a grocery list and prep for the week. This will save you time and money!
- Have fun searching for recipes. To add some variety to your menu, try new ones! Being healthy is a positive so have fun with it! Your meal planning is adjustable, so you do not have to feel boxed in.
- When you meal prep, do not feel like you have to do everything in one day. You can cut your vegetables one day, and make your sauces on the next day. You can also, go ahead and prepare the ingredients, even the spices you are going to use beforehand so the cooking will be seamless.
-

Quick Meal Plan Ideas

Breakfast

- Salmon cakes, arugula salad, and oranges.
- Loaded veggie sweet potato with kale, tomatoes, red beans, baby spinach, and green and red peppers.
- Spicy fruit medley with strawberries, watermelon, cantaloupe, pineapple sprinkled with brown sugar and a smidgen of red pepper.
- Cinnamon banana pancakes and baby spinach.
- Fried egg over a salad, tomato or wilted kale.
- Overnight oats with almond milk and your favorite fruits and vegetables.
- Quinoa with cinnamon and pineapple drizzled with a little agave or honey.

Lunch

- Taco bowl with beans, lettuce, tomatoes, avocado, and salsa.

- Rainbow salad with every color of fruit and vegetable on it.
- Pita bread pizza with tomato sauce, cheese, and your favorite meat topping.
- Salmon salad and fruit.
- Black bean, cabbage, and cheese quesadilla.
- Spaghetti and meatballs with mushrooms and green peppers, blueberries and salad.
- Fish, white beans, and coleslaw.

Dinner

- Veggie lasagna, and steamed broccoli.
- Breakfast veggies and eggs scramble.
- BLT with a side salad.
- Bean burgers and potato skins.
- Teriyaki chicken stir fry.
- Salisbury steaks and sweet potatoes.
- Chicken noodle soup and toasted cheese bread.

If you are considering going vegetarian or vegan for maximum benefits, here are a few common substitutions that you will want to know.

- For dairy milk, you can substitute any type of non-dairy milk like almond milk, soy milk or cashew milk. You can also make your own milk by soaking cashews in water overnight and then blending the cashews with water and adding extracts like vanilla or almond or whichever you prefer to give it extra flavor.
- For recipes that require yogurt, you can look into substituting a vegan alternative for yogurt.
- Butter, mayonnaise, cheese or cream cheese can be substituted for any vegan brand of the same product
- There are many different ways to substitute eggs. You

can use tofu instead of eggs if you're looking for a scrambled texture. If you're using eggs to bind items in a recipe, you can use unsweetened applesauce, soft tofu, mashed bananas or the popular flax seed egg, which is just 1 tablespoon of ground flax seeds plus 3 tablespoons of water or another liquid and blend it all together. Then add the flax egg to the recipe.

- For meaty textures, you can try tofu. Use seitan or meatless meat. You can also use mushrooms or cauliflower, instead of meat, or even blended nuts to give it the same meaty texture.
- Instead of using honey, you can use agave, maple syrup, or any type of plant-based sweetener.
- There are also many different types of fish substitutions. You can search for your favorite vegan fish substitute to still enjoy fish recipes.

Don't be afraid to create your own meal plans. You can even visit popular websites online, and they can give you popular meal plans for free. It will save you time and money in the long run. The next pillar you need to remember is exercise.

Exercise

To determine the best exercise regimen for your newfound lifestyle, it is best to think about what your body type, or somatype, is. There are three main body types: an endomorph, an ectomorph, and a mesomorph. Most people are not categorized in a single category - they are a combination of 2 or 3 of the body types. By knowing what type of body type you have is the first step towards getting healthier.

An endomorph body type is usually considered big-boned. Endomorphs normally gain weight very easily. They are typically short, stocky, and round. No matter what they do, it can seem very difficult to lose weight. The next body type is called a mesomorph. These are the people that can eat whatever they want and seem never to gain any weight. Oh yeah, they never work out either, and they do not gain any weight. Why is that? It is because their bodies already have a high metabolism and the blessed gift of genetics. While it seems like mesomorphs do not have anything to worry about in regard to weight loss, there is a downside. Because mesomorphs are naturally gifted with thinner figures, some do not take care of their bodies or eat the way that they should. Thus, when it is time for them to live a healthier lifestyle, it can become difficult for them to form healthy habits.

An ectomorph would essentially be in the middle of an endomorph and a mesomorph. An ectomorph doesn't have as much have trouble losing weight like an endomorph, but they can have trouble putting on muscle if they aren't strategic in how they build their weight. If you are an endomorph, it is best to do high interval training, cardio exercise. If you are an ectomorph, you can do cardio, but you will want to incorporate weight lifting as well. And if you are a mesomorph a combo of cardio and weight lifting is ideal. Again, your goals will help you determine which exercise regime is best. No matter what exercise you do, it is recommended that you get at least 30 minutes of active exercise every day or 150 minutes a week to keep your heart healthy.

If you do not have money for a gym membership or personal trainer, one of the easiest ways to get a workout in, is to look for exercise routines online, especially on YouTube. There are a lot of free workouts on there. If you are sedentary most of the time and have a little extra money to spend, you can invest in a desk peddler or a standing desk so you can move while you are working.

Another quick way to work out is just to do those basic old-fashioned exercises that you used to do in grade school, such as push-ups, sit-ups, jumping rope, and jumping jacks for thirty minutes. However, the key to this type of workout is to go as fast as you can and perform the exercises in sets. Perhaps you can do 3 sets of one exercise, rest, then do another three set of exercises and rest and keep going until you reach your 30 minutes. Exercise is something you definitely want to incorporate into your intermittent lifestyle if you want to maintain results and if you want to live in overall health or life. Do not make excuses. Find a way to be active!

Routine

Of course, when you first start off intermittent fasting, you may take some time to get adjusted. Get into a routine as soon as you can. If you need a little extra support, do not be afraid to look into health apps that offer health coaching. That may just be the extra boost you need. Health apps are truly popular and growing every day. You will be sure to find one that you need as long as you do a quick search on the App Store. A quick note. If you are doing an extended fast for over three days, you will want to go easy on the exercise.

Sleep

Lastly, sleep is going to be integral to your intermittent fasting journey. As mentioned before, if you are not sleeping well, you do not want to start intermittent fasting. Sleep helps your body handle the rigors of intermittent fasting and should not be overlooked. Try to get more sleep. If we do not get enough sleep, that's when you begin to compensate with unhealthy eating choices.

Sleeping is very important to a healthy lifestyle. This is one area where you do not want to skimp on. Give yourself seven to eight hours a night and watch the difference it will have in your life. Your mood will improve, your weight will improve, and your productivity will improve. Sleeping is underrated. Give it a try and watch how it affects your life. If you don't sleep, be prepared to suffer the consequences. This is not written to scare you, but to let you know that if you are serious about intermittent fasting and your health, these are four pillars that you will not overlook.

Give yourself a round of applause because we are almost at the end of the book. This book gave you the most important pillars you should have established in your life if you want to succeed with intermittent fasting long-term. The next chapter is all about the tips you need in order to be successful in your intermittent fasting journey. These tips include a lot of great practical steps that will help you overcome even the fiercest hunger pains.

Chapter 9: Tips to Help You Along the Way

As you continue to intermittent fast, you will notice that some days are easier than others, and some days are harder than others. The tips in this chapter are written to help you stay the intermittent fasting path and get the most out of your intermittent fasting journey, so every day is a good day.

First of all, when intermittent fasting, **listen to your body**. When you are eating, do not overeat. If you are full, do not keep eating. Your body will let you know when it has had enough. When you first begin intermittent fasting, it is expected that you will have hunger pangs. Your stomach may grumble here and there, and you may experience a headache, especially if you are used to eating and drinking a lot of sugar and caffeine. That is why what you eat is important.

Please note that if your hunger pangs turn into diarrhea, severe cramps or vomiting or any extreme type of symptoms, be sure to reach out to your healthcare professional. However, most hunger pangs can be avoided or prevented by eating nutrient-dense foods during meal times to help you make it through your fasting windows. Again, it is expected to take your time to adjust to your first intermittent fasting period, but after a week or two, you should feel more energized and well rested than before. So, what types of food should you be consuming?

You want to eat **whole foods that contain lots of macronutrients**. Macronutrients you want in your food include carbohydrates, fat, protein, minerals, vitamins, and water. I also want to make fiber an honorable mention. When you eat food with high levels of fiber, your digestive health improves. A simple rule of thumb is to keep your plate with as many varied colors as possible. Foods to consider eating are going to be lots of leafy vegetables like kale, swiss chard, greens, and lettuce; dark fruit like blackberries, raspberries, and strawberries, and drink lots of water even if you are already drinking lots of water. You can look into getting protein from non-meat sources such as nuts, quinoa or beans.

Do not forget to **avoid worthless calories or foods that do not contain many nutrients** that will keep you full, especially foods with lots of sugar. Sugar is everywhere! It is one of the most difficult things to cut out of your diet. However, if you want intermittent fasting to work, you will definitely want to be diligent against sugar. An ingredient to look for would be ingredients that end in 'ose' or anything that says, 'high fructose corn syrup.' Easy ways to give up sugar is to gradually get rid of them by eliminating the most obvious culprits that have a high sugar count such as candy, soda (diet or otherwise), or juice.

Also, **giving up carbohydrates** helps you rid yourself of the sugar. By eating whole foods with a dense nutrient count, it will help you avoid those cravings until you no longer even want sugar. While alcohol is not forbidden, it is one of those foods that take up calories without giving you many nutrients in return. Be mindful of those sneaky sugar calories in workout drinks or salty post-workout snacks that do not really help you enjoy the benefits of your workout! Additionally, when you go out to eat, try to have a peek at the menu in advance and try to pick out the options that fit into your calorie count.

One of the major keys to surviving any fasting period is the importance of **staying hydrated**. It also helps you not enter starvation mode. Of course, you will want to drink water, but there are other liquids, you should be aware of. The key to drinking while fasting is to partake in drinks that have no calories. Here's a list of drinks you should consider drinking while fasting.

- **Water** - Water is one of the best liquids to consume while fasting. You can add a slice of lemon or infuse it with herbs, like basil, mint, or your favorite fruit. It is important to stay away from any sweeteners that can mess up your fast. This means you want to avoid sugary water enhancers like Crystal Light or any type of artificial flavoring to give the water more flavor. Enjoy the water as I,s and let it help you make it through the fast. To make your water fancier, you may even want to consider sparkling water. Mineral water is also great to drink during your fast.
- **Broth** - Any type of vegetable or bone -flavored broth can help you make it through a fast. If you can, you want to stay away from the store-bought broth that will have lots of extra sodium and flavors the best thing to do is to make your own broth. The broth is really helpful when you are fasting for longer than 24 hours.
- **Tea** - Any type of tea has proved to be extremely beneficial when you are fasting. Oolong, herbal, black, and green tea are all great to drink while you are fasting. Generally, tea improves your gut digestion, cellular detox, and balance of your probiotics. Be sure to watch the caffeine intake with the teas. It's good to go for caffeine-free options like ginger, chamomile, lemongrass, and hibiscus. You don't want to get

addicted to caffeine or use it too much tea as an appetite suppressant while you are fasting.

Peppermint tea helps get rid of your bloating and gas. Cinnamon chai tea is great to bust any sugar cravings you may have. Oolong and black tea lower your blood sugar. Lastly, green tea is great for an appetite suppressant.

- **Apple cider vinegar** -This is another type of liquid that can be very helpful during your fasting period as it helps improve your digestion and can help suppress your appetite.
- **Coffee** - Another great liquid to have during your fast is coffee. If you drink coffee, you want to make sure it does not cause an upset stomach or cause a racing heart. If drinking coffee does this to you, you may consider not drinking it. When drinking coffee in your fast, you also want to avoid using any artificial sweeteners, milk, or cream that will add extra calories. Avoid butter and coconut oil, too.

If you want to flavor your coffee, consider adding spices like cinnamon, nutmeg or ginger for the bowl people.

- **Smoothies** - Smoothies are another great way to get the nutrition that you need. You can add vegetables to get the most out of your diet.
- **Pureed Soups** - These are great as well. You can even consider pureeing your favorite low-calorie meal if you want to stick to the liquid fast. This is another way you can get the nutrients that you need.

Now for the bad. Drinks you want to stay away from including sugary sodas, coconut water, juices, workout drinks like Gatorade or Powerade and definitely energy drinks. Almond milk is also a beverage you want to avoid while fasting. All these drinks have extra calories which will null-and-void your fast.

One more important thing to know about liquids is that it can help you beat symptoms of hunger while you are fasting. If you are having issues with dizziness or headaches, you will want to drink more water. Mineral water is also great for both of these issues. If you are having muscle cramps, you will want to drink water and soak in an Epsom salt bath to soak in. You may also consider taking a magnesium supplement. Lastly, if you are experiencing constipation, eat more fiber and drink more water during your eating period. You'll want to have more fruits, vegetables, and even chia seeds that have been soaked in a liquid like almond milk or even water if you're watching your calories.

Short-Term Strategies

When you are hungry, you want to eat immediately. You do not have time to think about long-term solutions to your hunger. You need something fast and efficient to help you cope so you can make it through your fasting window. The strategies in this section will help you do just that. These strategies are intended to help you with the here and now. Make a note of the ones you think that are specifically helpful. Choose 1 to 3 methods to lean on as you begin to help you cope with your hunger. You can play around with the different methods until you figure out which ones are the best for you.

- Eat a small snack. If you do eat a snack, go for a snack that under 50 calories and low-fat. If you must snack, make sure you include them in your meal planning efforts.
- Immediately distract yourself by playing a video game or another distraction to help you keep your mind off the hunger. If video games are not your thing, try to get distracted by pleasurable activities, especially ones that burn calories like taking a jog around the neighborhood or calling and speaking with a friend.
- Tap into the power of smell and smell something that smells like jasmine or vanilla. Both are shown to help crave sugar cravings.
- Take a nap. Sometimes hunger is an indication of being tired, not being hungry. The next time you are hungry, take a quick nap and see if the hunger resides once you wake up. Worst case scenario, the nap will serve as a distraction from your hunger and you will wake up not feeling hungry at all.
- When that hunger pang hits, floss and brush your teeth. You can even put a minty lip chap on with the hopes of the mint stopping you from getting too hungry. You can also pop a strong mint like an Altoid. The mint flavor should encourage you not to eat and mess up the freshness of your breath.
- Take a deep breath or do a few quick yoga poses to help clear your mind, and stop your cravings.
- When you eat, make sure you're chewing at least 30 times before you swallow. This makes sure that you are properly digesting your food, enjoying the flavors and slowing down your meal to make sure you are not overeating.
- When your next craving hits, take the time to do for tea. Make a fancy tea time with a cup of hot tea. You

can also do a nice cup of ginger tea as ginger has been shown to help stop cravings. Avoid sugary pastries and sweeteners during this tea time. You can also try fancy infused water, with mint, pomegranate, basil or cucumber or your favorite fruits instead. If tea or water isn't your thing, just do coffee instead. Remember, to limit the sweeteners and try to drink everything without creamer or sugar.

- Using acupuncture techniques is another way to try and curb your hunger. Tap your forehead for 30 seconds or try pinching your earlobes and nose.
- Another popular remedy to curbing your hunger is to chew gum, especially

after lunchtime. Chewing gum can help you make it to your next eating window. Be sure to go for the sugarless variety. If you notice that you have any stomach issues after chewing gum for long periods of time, select a different, hunger coping mechanism.

- Consider avoiding snacks. There have been people to say that snacking throughout the day is helpful for losing weight. The truth is that the total number of calories determine whether if you lose weight. So if you are a snacker and you need them to function, continue to do so as long as the snack does not interfere with your daily calorie count. However, try to take them out and just eat the main meals during your eating period to see if you notice a difference or not.
- When you eat, make sure you are chewing at least 30 times before you swallow. This makes sure that you are properly digesting your food, enjoying the flavors and slowing down your meal to make sure you are not

overeating.

- Also, stop eating a little bit before you feel complete and drink water. This is another good tip to help you prevent overeating.
- Next, try not to sleep after you eat. This won't help you as you try to become more efficient with fasting. It will actually hinder your progress.
- Drink lots of water and do not forget to take your vitamins. Water is an important way to intermittent fast successfully.
- Use your imagination and let yourself give in mentally. Imagine yourself eating whatever you want as a way to satisfy your hunger.
- Think about how eating your craving will affect you in the future. Will eating bring you closer or further away from your goals. Thinking of the long-term effects of not sticking to your fast may prevent you from eating during the fasted state.
- Just ignore the hunger pains. They typically last for 15 minutes. They come in bursts. If you can hold off for 15 minutes, you should be home free.
- Take a spoonful of apple cider vinegar after you eat or even before a meal. If you take it after you eat, the apple cider will help you make it through your fasted window. If you take the apple cider vinegar before you eat, it can help curb your appetite before you eat. If you take a spoonful while you are hungry, it can help you make it through your intermittent fasting window.
- The worst case scenario is just to give in and eat. Eat a very small portion, chew slowly and enjoy it. If you really give in, try to forgive yourself. We aren't always perfect, and sometimes we have to eat. However, try

to go without eating for as long as you can before you give in. Try not to make it a habit.

Long-Term Strategies

The strategies in this section aim to help you create habits that will help you long term on your intermittent fasting journey. Depending on your personality and your budget, these strategies can be easy or more difficult to implement. These strategies are ones that you should try once you have figured out that you are committed to being an intermittent faster. Even if you are not committed after you give it a test drive, some of these methods will still help you monitor your food intake. Ideally, your goal should be to incorporate these tips and let them become a habit to help to make intermittent fasting for your easier.

- Try to coordinate your intermittent fasting with your schedule you are already following. Keep in mind that after about five hours, unless you are sleeping overnight, your blood sugar levels drop and you begin to crave food. If you can craft your fasting and eating windows with this concept in mind, it will be easier with you to deal with your hunger.
- Try to avoid purchasing high fructose corn syrup, because it is an additive.

If you eat something with high fructose corn syrup in it, you will tend to want more of it. If you want some, it can cause you to want more. Other names high fructose syrup go by includes: fructose, maize syrup, glucose syrup, fructose or glucose syrup, tapioca syrup, fruit fructose, crystalline fructose or HFCS. Anytime you see one of these names your intermittent fasting antennae should be up and you should try and avoid that food.

- Next, try to avoid eating refined sugar which is often found in white sugar, white flour or white pasta. Try to replace it with natural sweeteners, nut flours, or whole grain pasta or forgo these ingredients all together.
- Purchase blue plates for your home. Blue plates are shown to help prevent cravings. This may be a little pricey so do not be afraid to check second-hand stores for this item. Also, try using smaller plates that will help limit your portions sizes. Using bigger forks can also make you feel fuller in a shorter amount of time.
- Try to get more sleep. If we do not get enough sleep, that's when you can

begin trying to compensate with unhealthy eating choices. Sleeping is very important to a healthy lifestyle. This is one area where you do not want to skimp on. Give yourself seven to eight hours a night and watch the difference it will have in your life. Your mood will improve, your weight will improve, and your productivity will improve. Sleeping is underrated. Give it a try and watch how it affects your life.

- Create a list of items to do that calms you, makes you happy or that you enjoy. Try to let them be things that do not involve eating. Try to create 25 things and pick one the next time you are hungry pick one from the list.
- Are you an emotional eater? If so, try to get to the root cause of why you are eating when you are emotional. Remember that journal you were supposed to keep from earlier? Be sure to note any trends of when you

are eating if you are bored, stressed, sad, or mad, then adjust your behavior accordingly. Be mindful of what you are eating so you do not eat because you are bored or stressed.

- Just like hunting for high fructose syrup or refined sugars, get into the habit of reading food labels. You'll want to pay special attention to the serving size. This will help you not if you are overeating or not. Also, saturated fats and sodium are other categories that you want to pay attention to and choose foods that are high in fiber. When you add more fiber to your meal, it helps you make it through your fasting periods easier. You'll also want to pay special attention to the vitamins and minerals in the food to make sure it is full of good food for you.

- Make the lights brighter when you eat your meals. This is an interesting tip and may be on the pricey side if you need to buy a few new or brighter bulbs. Bright lights raise the awareness of what you are eating; whereas, dim lights tend to lower your inhibitions. This means when the lights are low, you tend to pig out. Keep those lights bright, so you do not overeat and effectively ruin your intermittent fasting eating window.

- Another quick way to help you watch what you eat and prevent you from pigging out during your window is to have a soup or salad as an appetizer first. You can also have a cup of water first. This tip can fill you up with good nutrients and help you not to overeat.

- Although it sounds counterintuitive, you will want to eat the same foods every day. This helps your body to adjust easier and helps make meal planning easier to make sure you are getting the proper nutrients and calories that you need.

If you are a person who believes that spice is the variety of life, do not be afraid to try new things after at least eating a set schedule for a few days to see how your body reacts. The best to back your diet is with foods that are bulky but low in calories like whole grains, beans, fruits, and vegetables.

Whether you are interested in adding short-term or long-term strategies to your life, both of these categories can help you make it when you feel like your stomach is going to fall through your back. Again, pick one to two strategies to start with, and note them in your food journal. You will be able to track and see which methods work the best for you and which ones are keepers and which ones you need to replace.

If you are still not convinced that you are able to overcome your hunger, then this next section is for you. If you want to curb your hunger, there are just some foods that are better to eat than others. These foods help you make it through your fasting periods with ease because they can suppress your appetite due to their ingredients. Do not be afraid to add these ingredients to your shopping list.

- **Eggs** - There is nothing like starting your day off with a hard-boiled egg. This helps you make it to lunchtime because it is packed with protein. Increasing other methods of protein can help you keep your hunger satisfied for longer.
- **Coffee** – This is another great way to start your day because it is an appetite suppressant. Coffee, if you

can take it no sugar or sweetener, is a great beverage to add to your intermittent fasting schedule. You can opt for green tea if coffee isn't your thing. You can add cinnamon, cloves or ginger to either hot drink because these grounds spices help lower your blood sugar levels which help you keep your appetite under control.

- **Cayenne pepper or any type of spicy** pepper - If you are not used to spicy food, adding a little spice to your meals will help you control your hunger. Although its counterintuitive, many people in hot countries known for spicy foods use this exact method of control their appetites so they won't feel lethargic in the hot sun from eating heavy meals. Adding hot sauce is another alternative if you can't tolerate spice. Tabasco or sriracha sauce are all great options.

- **Almonds** – Almonds are considered one of those healthy fats that can help you go longer without eating. If you do not like almonds, try your favorite nut instead. For an extra boost, you can look into creating your own trail mix by combining granola dark chocolate dried fruit in your favorite nuts. You can season the mixture with a little pepper or ginger to give them an extra kick. This protein-packed snack will definitely Chris your hunger and help you make it through your intermediate fasting windows.

- **Dark Chocolate** – Dark chocolate is healthier than milk chocolate, and it is a good way to help suppress your hunger while giving you a taste of sweetness to help satisfy your sweet tooth. For vegans, don't be afraid to try being chocolate. It may be a pleasant surprise.

- **Grapefruit** – This fruit is a popular option to have as a snack because it lowers your insulin, and helps you lost weight. Also, there are different types of grapefruit that you can try. Expand your palate and find a grapefruit that you like and take advantage of the macronutrients that it has.

- **Lots of magnesium** – Any dark green, leafy vegetable like kale, charge, or spinach are going to be great for you to help suppress your appetite for longer periods of time. If you want to down your greens all at one time, blend them together in a smoothie with your favorite beverage. You can add a healthy sweetener or some fruit to give it a little sugar to make the drink go down easier. Drinking a smoothie when you are hungry like this is extremely helpful and make sure that you reach your daily nutrient vegetable quote. If you're worried about your caloric content, it's okay. You can never have enough vegetables.
- **Skim milk** – This is especially useful if women drink a glass a day for about a week or two before their periods. The milk helps women control their cravings, so they do not binge once their menstrual cycle comes.
- **Sushi** – The wasabi paste in sushi is a great way to help suppress your appetite. Sushi is also a healthy low-calorie snack to eat. Tofu, which contains genistein, that helps you eat less and stay full longer is also a great ingredient to add to your daily food plan. Another Asian ingredient, umeboshi plums, which can be found at your local Asian grocer is sour and an appetite suppressant which is excellent for dealing with sugar cravings.
- **Water** – If you drink this before every meal, it is a sure-fire way to help you not overeat. Exercising before your major meal of the day is another way to

help suppress your appetite.

- **Yerba Mate tea** – This tea helps to reduce your appetite and helps improve your mood. It is in the same category as ginger tea. Do not overlook taking advantage of this drink.
- **Protein-rich and healthy-fat foods** – Avocados, lean meats, nuts, and cheese are very helpful to eat.
- **Oats** – They are full of fiber, cheap, and help you feel fuller for longer periods.
- **Jacket Potatoes** – The skin on potatoes are full of fiber. If you pack the potatoes with veggies, the benefits of eating it will last longer. If you use sweet potatoes, this only ups the ante.
- **Your favorite smoothie** – If you have a veggie jam-packed with a scoop of protein or your favorite whey protein, you will beat able to combat hunger. This helps you meet your daily veggie dietary needs and helps you keep your appetite in check.

Learning to overcome your hunger is no joke. It is a very real concern that many people have before they begin intermittent fasting. The good news is that there are short-term strategies and long-term strategies that can help you overcome any hunger pains you may have. The more your body gets used to your fasting windows, the easier it will be to make it through them. Overcoming hunger is mental as well as physical. If you are eating a well-balanced diet, being consistent and are determined to make it work, you will. As you intermittent fast, make sure that you are paying close attention to your cravings.

Giving in to Cravings

We all get hungry, but some of us never pay attention to what we are craving for at the moment. In order to survive, our bodies want certain nutrients, vitamins, and minerals to sustain us. Sometimes, we just want good ol' water. The following section details what our cravings could be telling us. When you are writing in your food journal, pay special attention to what you are craving and what days. Noting the time and if you are craving these foods after any certain activities will also provide insight into what you are craving.

Keeping careful track of your cravings can help you figure out what you are craving and, in some cases, why. It will help you take your combatting hunger to another level. By focusing on what your hunger is telling you, you are making sure you are meeting your dietary needs as well as possibly catching any disturbing signals that your body may be telling you. Sometimes our bodies give similar signals for certain cravings, but the best thing to do if you are not sure what to do is to drink water. It typically helps with cravings and satiates hunger. Do not underestimate the power of paying attention to what your body is telling you. Listen and watch your body reward you for it.

Salty food

This is a good indicator that you need to drink more water. Our body responds to being dehydrated by craving salty foods. This is a common craving people have. If you have it, let an 8-ounce cup of water sooth it. Along with water, increase your intake of calcium, magnesium, and zinc. Make sure that you are not experiencing exhaustion, extreme weight loss or a change in the color of your skin. This could point to a larger health issue if you are craving salt all the time. To encourage you to drink more water, you can purchase a cool water bottle or personalized one that you already have to your liking. This will give a special touch to your water drinking. If you are a person who despises water, see if you can start with sugarless sparkling water or invest in sparkling water machine to make your own sparkling water at home. You can also consider infusing the water with different fruits to give it a taste. There are no ways around not drinking water. You just have to find a way to cope with drinking it that is to your liking.

Sweets

Just like salty foods, sugar craving is a good indicator that you need to drink more water. This craving is also related to your caffeine intake and your sleeping schedule. A sugar craving can also be your body's way to stay energized. So if you down lots of caffeine and barely are getting any sweets, try to get some sleep and lay off the caffeine as well. Another way to help ease this craving is to incorporate more naturally sweet fruits and vegetables into your diet, like carrots, sweet potatoes, beets, apples or vegetables into your diet. Instead of sugar, you can try natural sweeteners such as agave or maple syrup instead of sugary snacks and drinks. Honey is touted as helping you feel full longer so do not overlook this favorite sweetener or many. If you are always craving something sweet, try something sour to kill the craving. Sour foods also help improve your digestive system. Lastly, incorporating more protein in your diet can also help you overcome the sugary diet as your body will be sustained and you do not have to rely on sugar to pick your body up.

Chocolate, cheese, and dairy products

If you are craving chocolate or cheese, you may need to pick up your mood. Chocolate and cheese are known as comfort foods and rightfully so since they release feel-good chemicals to improve your mood. If you notice that you are having these types of cravings, look for ways to boost your mood like taking a quick jog or doing a few quick stretches at your desk. If you are still struggling with chocolate and dairy cravings after trying to improve, you can consider looking into vegan options or eliminating it from your diet altogether. Ridding themselves of dairy has helped a lot of people with their health journey, and if you do that on your intermittent fasting path, you may be surprised at the results.

Ice or red meat

This could point to an iron deficiency. If you have low iron, increase your protein intake or even eat more red meat. If you are vegan or vegetarian, see about increasing your intake with beats of plant-based sources or protein. Make sure this craving is not coupled with any drastic skin or hair changes, as well. Iron is an important aspect of a healthy lifestyle, so don't overlook this craving if you have it.

Soda

Craving a carbonated, sugary soda suggests that you may have a calcium deficiency. Increase your calcium intake to help with this craving. You can find calcium in leafy green vegetables if you are vegan and other plant-based sources so do not feel that you only can find calcium in dairy. If you are craving the carbonation so you can burp, try sparkling water or club soda with fruit infused in it to see if it will give you that same field. Sparkling water is a much healthier option than soda, and it gives you some of the same joys of burping that soda does.

French fries and potato chips

A craving such as this means that you need to eat more healthy fats found in oily fish like salmon, sardines or nut. If this is a persistent craving, you should also consider adding more fiber, magnesium and chromium food that is found in foods like chard, celery, spinach, apricots, apples, and bananas. If you just can't seem to rid yourself of the potato chip or French fry craving, create your own healthier options from sweet potatoes or white potatoes. You can also thinly slice some vegetables and create your own crunchy vegetables by roasting them with a little extra virgin olive oil in the stove. These are some healthier alternatives, and you may become addicted to them just like you are to French fries and chips, which would not be a bad problem to have.

Any other cravings

Drink more water to try to help the craving. Also, note if you can tell any weird other things happening with your bodies such as extreme weight loss or weird mood swings or any other dramatic changes. Some food cravings can point to pregnancy if you are a woman or other health issues for men and women. Always err on the side of caution. If you feel like something weird is going on, trust your instincts. Health Care Providers are there for a reason. Don't be afraid to reach out to them.

If you are eating a well-balanced diet, then your craving issues should be easier to manage and control. Not just a well-balanced diet, but drinking a lot of water is helpful, too. The next section will focus on the best foods to eat to help you not have such severe cravings. Now the part that we've all been waiting for is the next section. This section will help you eat the best foods that can help you control your hunger throughout the day. This last section will focus on what to do if you feel like your body is plateauing at any moment.

Plateauing

After you start fasting, you may run into a few issues. You have lost a couple of pounds, but now you are not sure how to lose more. You've seemed to flatline. What do you do next? This section is all about how to maintain the weight you have lost and how to overcome any ruts you may run into.

First things first, here are a few questions to ask yourself about how to maintain your weight. When you initially start intermittent fasting, you may see huge results, but if at any time you begin to eat more and not exercise portion control, there is the chance you may gain that weight back. However, there are some ways to try and monitor your weight so you can stay on the straight-and-narrow intermittent path.

- When you look in your food journal or your calorie are you still eating the same amount of calories? Has that number changed at all? If so, why? And how can you fix it? What other weird trends do you notice? For example, on days that you are busy, you notice that you always break your fast? How can you fix some of the challenges on the trends that you see?
- Are you drinking enough water? Sometimes you are not hungry, you are dehydrated and drinking more water can prevent you from eating worthless calories.
- When are you eating? Are you using eating to cope with any emotional issues you may be having? Are you emotional eating for fun or to deal with any sadness? Paying attention to when you are eating can help you nip emotional eating in the bud.
- Are you binging during your meals when you can eat or are you eating normal potions? It is expected that you may gain some weight back if you are eating double portions to compensate for when you are not eating. The idea is to keep the same amount of food that you are eating so your body can reap the benefits of a true fasting period.
- Additionally, what types of foods are you eating? Has the method you chose fit easily into your current lifestyle or are you having a difficult time fasting with the current method you've chosen. Are you only

eating carbohydrates like bread and pasta with limited fruits and vegetables? If you must have some of your favorite unhealthy foods, see if you can find a vegetarian or vegan or a healthier version of that recipe.

- Have you tried a different fasting window? A different window can sometimes provide better results. You can play around with different fasting windows until you find the one that works the best for you.
- How is your sugar intake? Are you still eating sugar in high amounts or even eating foods that have those sneaky sugar calories hidden inside them? A review of the ingredients in the foods that you eat can help you find the culprit.
- Who's encouraging you? Are your friends and family being supportive or negative Nancys?
- Are there any days where you are feeling dizzy, nauseated, fatigued or having difficulty concentrating? What are the foods that you are eating when you notice these symptoms? This will help you figure out if the food you are eating is agreeable or if you need to eat more or less of certain foods.
- Do you have any cravings? At what time? What are you doing on the days that you are having cravings?
- Are your meals well-balanced? Are you seeing a lot of different colors from different food groups on your plate when you eat or only one type of color?
- How fast did you transition to intermittent fasting? Are you getting enough calories for your energy needs? If you are drastically below the recommended count for women or men, you may need to eat more.
- Are you eating enough when you work out? Are you carb cycling (which means you eat a slightly bigger portion on your workout days versus the days when

you do not workout)?

- Are you having trouble binging on sugar or having a difficult time breaking bad habits? If so, perhaps you can allow yourself at least 3 cheat meals a month to satisfy those cravings.
- What type of exercises are you doing? Are the exercises complementary to weight or muscle gain? If the exercises you are doing are helping you gain muscle, like lifting weights, you may not be losing weight, but you are gaining muscle which can help you lose weight in the long term. More cardio based exercises can help you burn more calories and potentially lose more weight. Be sure to make sure your exercise regimen is helping you reach your goals.

Mind you, if you were to stop at all, you might gain some of the weight that you've lost. So keep going! Do not give up. The race is not to the swift but to those who endure, be mindful that you may not see changes because you are with your body all the time. However, if you ask someone else, they may be able to point out changes that you are not aware of so do not be afraid to ask for a second opinion. Stay positive!

Additionally, weight loss may not be the first benefits you see. Note your mood and your focus and your energy levels to see if intermittent fasting has made an impact on your life in other ways besides wait. Trust me, people will know and talk about it if they notice a difference. If they don't, that's okay too. Just ask for their honest opinion and see what they have to say if you need some validation. Just make sure the person that you're asking if someone that you trust and who has your best interest in mind.

Remember, if you do not see your expectations being met as quickly as you expect, it is okay to make a few changes to see if you can reach your goals. After tweaking a few things while you fast and still aren't meeting your expectations, it may be time to get more realistic ones. Nevertheless, keep working with your intermittent fasting windows, your meal, and portion choices as well as your exercise routines until you get the results that you want. Mistakes and mishaps are inevitable, but it is important to keep a good sense of humor and a sense of determination so you can make it through. Hopefully, this chapter has put to rest any fear that you may have about intermittent fasting and assured you of the benefits that it has. Even if you do not decide to stick with intermittent fasting long-term, at least giving it a try will open your eyes to a new method of living and your body will thank you.

Hopefully, you are convinced about all the benefits of intermittent fasting. Good luck on your journey!

Conclusion

Thank for making it through to the end of The Easy Intermittent Fasting for Women: The Ultimate Beginners Guide for Permanent Weight Loss, Burn Fat in Simple, Healthy, and Scientific Ways, and Heal Your Body Through the Self- Cleansing Process of Autophagy." Let's hope it was informative and able to provide you with all of the tools you need to achieve your goals whatever they may be.

Intermittent fasting is not new to humankind. From the beginning of time up until today, the benefits of intermittent fasting have been lauded by philosophers and health practitioners alike. Some of the earliest indications of the benefits of fasting were to deal with sickness. Researchers today have shown that intermittent fasting is indeed healthy, and it has many health benefits that can help you live a long and healthy life. For Americans who are dealing with unhealthy lifestyles, intermittent fasting may just be the solution that they are looking for. The journey to intermittent fast name is an easy one to start, but maintaining it can be difficult. Whether you are afraid of not being able to make it through your fat and window or just afraid that your body will go haywire once you begin, these, along with all other valid concerns, can be overcome if you do a slow and gradual approach to intermittent fasting.

Just as a bonus tidbit, there are many celebrities who follow the intermittent fasting lifestyle with wonderful results. You are not the only person who knows the value of intermittent fasting. Celebrities have long been practicing intermittent fasting for years. Check out who they are and which fasting style works best for them.

- Jimmy Kimmel follows the 5:2 intermittent dieting. It has helped him maintain his weight. For him, he eats about 500 calories every Thursday and Monday. On the other days, he eats what he wants. But, guess what? He drinks on the days that he's fasting. Yup, good ol' coffee to help him make it through the day.
- Terry Crews typically eats from 2-10 pm every day. He follows the 16:8 intermittent fasting lifestyle. He works out while fasting and feels like intermittent fasting has helped him stay in shape. He even sometimes eat a little coconut oil on a spoon to help him make it through his fast, a great tip to know. He also states that intermittent fasting has him feeling better than he was younger due to intermittent fasting's know energy boosting effects.
- Jennifer Metcalfe is another celebrity who follows the 5:2 intermittent fasting plan and notes how it helps her with her workouts and give her more energy as well.
- Hugh Jackman credits his intermittent fasting method of 16:8 as helping him maintain his weight. He also says that intermittent fasting helps him sleep well at night.
- Nicole Kidman is known to follow the 16:8 intermittent fasting method. She usually just eats lean proteins and lots of vegetables as well.
- Justin Theroux is an actor who cut out sugar and goes on about a 12 hour fast for about two to three weeks at a time. He eats from 7 am and 7 pm. He also drinks amino acids to help him curb his appetite.
- Beyoncé, although she has not confirmed due to her low-key profile, is also said to practice intermittent fasting.

- Chris Hemsworth has done the 15:9 method to lose weight for movies roles. He also eats 500-600 calories per day to lose for roles as a weight to get as most weight loss as possible by pairing intermittent fasting and a caloric deficit.
- Benedict Cumberbatch also does the 5:20 diet and eats less than 500 calories on his fasting days to maintain his physique for his movie roles.
- Ben Affleck, Jennifer Lopez, and Miranda Kerr are also known to practice intermittent fasting.

It seems like intermittent fasting is one of the best-kept secrets that stars use to get in shape for movie roles and to maintain their weight. Thankfully, you now know its value, and you can incorporate it in your life so you can be movie star ready as well.

The next step is to get started. It is my hope that you do not delay in starting your intermittent fasting lifestyle. The quicker you begin, the quicker you can start seeing improved health results and an improvement in overall health goals. So, how about you? What's holding you back? No more excuses.

The next step is to make a real commitment to start intermittent fasting. Decide what method you are going to use. Which window will fit best into your life as it is now? Would it be 5:3, 16:8, 12:12, or eat a day and skip a day, or even a two-week fast? Whichever one it is, pick that method, throw away all your junk food, make a meal plan, and get started! All the best! I cannot wait to see and hear all your wonderful stories! Soon, you will join the ends of people who know the power of intermittent fasting, and you will revel in the healthy your lifestyle that you now have thanks to the many benefits of an intermittent fasting lifestyle.

When you look back at the time that you were not intermittent fasting, you will be able to laugh and smile, knowing that you are now doing what you thought at one time was impossible. You will grin in the light in the fact that there is a sweetness in the stomach emptiness that you are now privy to enjoying.

Finally, if you found this book useful in any way, a review on Amazon is always appreciated!

CPSIA information can be obtained
at www.ICGtesting.com
Printed in the USA
LVHW082247180419
614770LV00029B/853/P